With Best Wishes
Ian C. Graham

AT THE STROKE OF ONE

BEFORE, DURING AND AFTER MY LIFE-CHANGING STROKE

IAN C GRAHAM

The Book Guild Ltd

First published in Great Britain in 2021 by
The Book Guild Ltd
9 Priory Business Park
Wistow Road, Kibworth
Leicestershire, LE8 0RX
Freephone: 0800 999 2982
www.bookguild.co.uk
Email: info@bookguild.co.uk
Twitter: @bookguild

Typeset in 11pt Minion Pro

Printed and bound in the UK by TJ Books LTD, Padstow, Cornwall

ISBN 978 1913551 957

British Library Cataloguing in Publication Data.
A catalogue record for this book is available from the British Library.

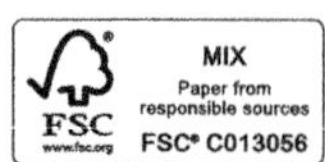

Dedication

I would like to dedicate this book to ALL the members of my Family, Friends, Sporting Colleagues, Work Colleagues and all who may have known me over the years.

I truly hope that you enjoy my writings, which I believe will give you a true insight into some of the happenings throughout my life.

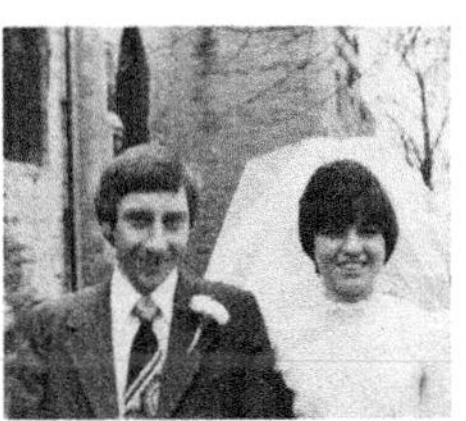

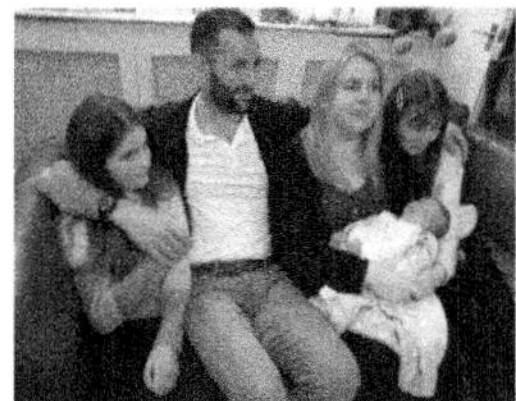

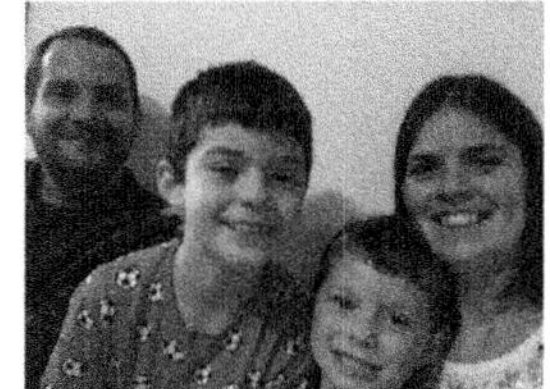

Dedication

I would like to dedicate this book to All the members of my Family, Friends, [illegible] Colleagues, Work Colleagues and all who may have [illegible] over the years.

Introduction

THE MONTH STARTED off well. Things couldn't have been much better if you had written a script.

Heather and I, along with our children Laura and Nicola, had succeeded in purchasing a hotel in Tintagel, North Cornwall – The Bossiney House Hotel. It was quite large, being a twenty-bedroom holiday hotel set in grounds of approximately 1.5 acres of mainly lawned gardens. Overlooking the North Cornwall coastline and the South West coastal path, the hotel was mainly frequented by the walking fraternity and enjoyed a quite large overseas agreement with a Germany-based company, Wikinger Reisen, who specialised in worldwide walking holidays.

Soon to join us – the following week, in fact – were Heather's parents, Pat and John Cannings, who had helped us financially to buy the business and had agreed to join us in Cornwall to work at the hotel with us, on a part-time basis. In reality they were joining us to semi-retire.

We were very pleased with ourselves and proud to be the new owners of such a large and prominent business and premises. In addition to the hotel, we had also purchased a three-bedroomed cottage and separate two-bedroomed flat as living accommodation, all of which were situated in the same grounds.

We arrived at the hotel on a Thursday evening in early May 1996, to find the hotel closed for business due to our impending takeover the following day. Our takeover was subject to the local magistrate's court at Bodmin granting us a temporary licence in respect of the hotel bar. The hearing for the licence transfer was due to take place the following morning, Friday 4th May 1996, at 10.00am.

When we arrived at the hotel on the Thursday evening we were met by the then current owners, Bob and Margaret Savage, along with their son David. Bob and Margaret were in partnership with Bob's brother Colin and his wife Sandra, who were already living at their new home in Treknow, a small village just outside Tintagel.

The first thing we did after being shown to our rooms for the night was to unload the Ford Galaxy that we had bought a couple of weeks earlier, in which we had travelled down from Yorkshire. Sophie, our Cavalier King Charles Spaniel, was first out, quickly followed by Flopsy the rabbit and then our pet goldfish, all of whom had survived the long journey, thankfully, surprisingly well.

Having been in the car for some seven hours, we were, as you would expect, quite hungry and very definitely thirsty. We were hoping that we would be able to eat at the hotel that evening, but as stated earlier, the hotel was completely closed pending our takeover the following day. Bob suggested that we eat at a local restaurant in Tintagel called The Riggs. After putting the luggage away in our rooms, we drove down to Tintagel for a very welcome meal.

I don't really know what we all expected of The Riggs, but I know that I fancied a nice large steak with all the trimmings.

When we arrived and looked at the menu, we found that the restaurant was really a snack-type establishment rather than what we were hoping for – a really nice restaurant! Little did I know what else was about to come…

Chapter 1

The Early Years

LIFE BEGAN FOR me in the early winter of 1949. Arriving on 7th January of that year in the village of Berry Brow in Huddersfield, West Yorkshire, I was the first of three children, all of us boys, to be born to Kathleen and Kenneth Graham, our much-loved parents. My first home was a back-to-back house with, as I seem to recall, only the one bedroom and situated just off a road called Deadmanstone Road. The area in my childhood and very early teens was to become my natural playground. My younger brother, Stephen, was also born at this house on 16th June 1951.

Living in the house at the rear of our house (theirs was the front house), lived George and Winnie Boothroyd. Uncle George and Auntie Winnie, they soon became and remained close to me for many years to come. In fact, Uncle George was to become quite an influence in my sporting life in later years, although quite naturally this was unbeknown to me at this time.

George was a local cricket professional with Huddersfield Cricket League side, Armitage Bridge, the next village to Berry Brow. This cricket club, and particularly the cricket field, was to become my inspiration in future years, to play this wonderful and extremely intriguing and typically British institutional game. George was also a well-known sporting gentleman, yes, gentleman, in Yorkshire and indeed was a goalkeeper with Huddersfield Town Football Club for a period in the 1940s. He later went on to play for Halifax Town and Bradford City among others.

In later years, after he had finished playing cricket and football, he became a very respected cricket umpire and football referee throughout the Huddersfield area, officiating in both capacities long after many people would have retired due to age catching them up. But not George – he loved his sport too much, and more so, the sport and people playing it loved George. He was that kind of man: honest, gentlemanly, respected and genuine, and looked up to by all who had the pleasure to know him in any way whatsoever.

I recall that the house enjoyed a rather large communal garden that was shared by the other three or four households in the terraced block. We had a shed in which the usual gardening tools and the like were kept and a rabbit hutch housing our rabbits. I don't remember much about them except that Mum and Dad used to let them out into the garden for exercise very often. At the right-hand end of the garden was a fairly large rock, almost like a cliff, at the top of which was situated Deadmanstone House.

This was a family-owned mansion house situated in quite large grounds. The local school were encouraged to hold their annual summer fete in the grounds and people used to come from miles around to enjoy what was usually a most enjoyable day with plenty to do for all ages. Local builders, Jack Brook Ltd, eventually purchased the house and grounds, and the whole area now affords a modern housing estate of traditional stone bungalows and dormer bungalows. Unsurprisingly the estate is known locally as the Deadmanstone Estate but officially as Wain Park.

There are a few legends that surround the unassuming eruption of rock in the hillside that may possibly explain how Deadmanstone became to be named.

Local folklore tells that in the days when the church at Almondbury served as the parish church for the Holme Valley, funeral processions passing the stone would stop and rest the coffin there. One such legend suggests that corpses would be taken from their coffins and pulled through the hole (cave in the rock) before recommencing on the journey to Almondbury.

Another suggests that the remains of a soldier, possibly from Roman times or maybe a victim of Scottish Border raiders, was found there. This legend isn't specific about where or when the soldier was found and could have been transposed from the site of Deadmanstone House or its medieval predecessor, which apparently was a fortified manor house with deep cellars. It could of course be something entirely different and we will probably never know how the area of Deadmanstone was derived. But I was born in the immediate locality!

At the edge of the estate still lies the Huddersfield to Sheffield railway line, which is not a main line these days but is still used regularly. At the other side of the railway was the local recreation ground ('Brow Rec), comprising of a football field, a play area with swings, slide and seesaw, and a reasonably large grassed area in which to play. Over the years this became a very popular meeting area and playground for most of us "Browers" when school was finished for the day and during the school holidays.

When I was about four years of age, my parents moved from Deadmanstone to Waingate, all of 300 yards away, and it was here that on 29th April 1955 my youngest brother, Glyn, was born. The house was number 18, which was situated in a block of terraced houses, some six or seven houses, as I recall. Also living in the block were my Grandma Berry (my mum's mother) and my Auntie Nellie (grandma's cousin). Apparently the three houses that we all lived in were owned by my grandma, whose husband Sam, who had passed away many years previously, had bought while he was a partner of a textile mill in Lockwood on the outskirts of Huddersfield. Had he lived, who knows what would be now?

Grandma Berry was born in 1903, married in 1923 and died in 1984. Grandad Berry, whom I obviously never knew, was born in 1891, married in 1923 and died in 1929, when my mother was just two years old. Effectively, she never really knew her father.

Aunt Nell was born in 1905, married in 1924 and died in 1975. She suffered from rheumatism and arthritis for many years and spent quite a lot of time in a hospital in Nottinghamshire that specialised in those areas. She married her husband Edgar, who was born in 1891, married in 1924 and died in 1952.

Whilst the houses were solidly built from natural stone, they were somewhat old and the floors on the ground floor were solid stone slabs. The ground floor consisted of the living room, which was situated at the front of the dwelling, and the kitchen at the rear. At the side of the kitchen was the coalhouse, or coalhole, as it was known in those days. For those readers who don't know what this was, it was where we stored the coal that was used for the heating of the house, and sometimes the cooking, as there was no such thing as central heating in those days!

On the first floor were of course two bedrooms. Both bedrooms faced the front of the house, with Mum and Dad sleeping in the slightly larger one of the two and Stephen and I in the other. The bathroom do I hear? Well, the bathroom for all of us was in the living room, in front of the fire, and consisted of a large tin bath, which had to be filled with buckets of hot water from the kitchen. As you can imagine, this took a fair amount of time, not to mention the effort involved. And the emptying of it – well!

Not to mention, the water had to be used by more than one of us, sometimes all of us.

No inside toilets either. If you needed to go you had two options. The toilet was situated in the back garden, which in our case required a short journey out of the front door (no back door), a walk through the passageway between our house (no. 18) and next door (no. 20), up about twenty steps, then a short walk to the rear of the garden and eventually, thank goodness, the loo! The other option was mainly used on a night and I leave this totally to your imagination.

We had a small dog at the time called Tess, who on a night, sometimes used to chase the rats that lived and scrounged around the Co-op buildings. She was quite adept at catching them, much to Dad's delight. In the passageway we also kept a hutch in which we kept three guinea pigs. Unfortunately, two of them were males and it didn't take all that long for them to fight, presumably over the female. Soon there were only two.

The rear garden was quite large, and whilst it wasn't used for growing vegetables or flowers and the like, it was a good playground for Stephen and me, along with a few friends. With the kitchens of the row of houses being at the back and of single-storey building, we were easily able to run across the kitchen roofs in both directions. Effectively we had a short cut to the areas that were situated behind Waingate. We had a lot of fun doing this, sometimes to the annoyance of the neighbours living there.

The houses were situated immediately opposite Berry Brow Co-operative Society. Having just about every department, selling almost everything that anyone in the village and surrounding area required, you did not need to travel into Huddersfield in order to buy anything much at all. The Co-op was situated in Waingate on the left side of the road when travelling down it. The office was situated at the top of the road, followed by a few houses and Kelly's Butchers, followed by the departments, all in separate but adjoining buildings. The cobblers, which also sold a large range of footwear, the greengrocers, where I was to work many years later, the butchers, the chemists and hardware shop, the grocery, the drapery and then a gap followed by a privately owned greengrocers and finally the Co-op Bakery.

At the rear of the Co-op buildings was the Coal Yard, also owned by the Co-op, which supplied coal to most of the residents in the area, as this was the main source of fuel for heating and sometimes cooking! All the departments were accessible to the rear by a small un-made road, by which replenishment supplies were delivered on a regular basis. Berry Brow Co-operative Society also owned the Netherton Co-operative Society situated approximately four miles away in the village of Netherton. They later acquired the Brockholes Co-operative Society, in another nearby village, after they ran into financial problems.

The village of Berry Brow must have been an extremely thriving village at this time, as it boasted a quite large variety of shops and businesses, etc. The following is a list of shops, businesses and licensed premises along with the owners, which was compiled by my mother during the late 1950s.

Sweet shop	Robin Hood Hill	J Cunnington
Golden Fleece Hotel	Robin Hood Hill	Unknown
Doctor's surgery	Parkgate	Dr Waddy (later Dr Garnet)
Fish and chip shop	Parkgate	Ainsworth's
Bread and confectionery	Parkgate	Mallinson's
Cycle shop	Parkgate	McCracken's
Confectioners	Parkgate	Beever's
Plumbers	Parkgate	Gledhill's
Butchers	Parkgate	Gledhill's
Bread and confectionary	Parkgate	J A Heeley
Berry Brow Liberal Club	Parkgate	Community
Sweet shop	Stockwell Hill	Spencer's

Post office and barbers	Stockwell Hill	Chas. Berry
Fish and chips then sweets	Stockwell Hill	A Brodie
Painters and decorators	Parkgate	Littlewood's
Chemists	Parkgate	Lomax's
Black Bull Hotel	Parkgate	Unknown
Hairdressers	Parkgate	Joyce Sanderson
Undertakers	Parkgate	Wilfred France
Butchers Arms Hotel	Parkgate	Unknown
Undertakers	Dodds Royd	John T Haigh
Papers and confectionery	Dodds Royd	M Haigh
Fish and chip shop	Waingate	Steads (later Roskell's)
Butchers	Waingate	Farrand (later Hinchliffe)
Sweet shop	Waingate	Wilf Cunnington
Joiner and undertakers	Waingate	Chas. Oldham
Drapery	Waingate	Cains
Cobblers	Waingate	Fred Hoyle
Grocers	Waingate	Scott Heeley
Grocery and confectionary	Bridge Street	J A Heeley
Sweet shop	Bridge Street	Midwood's
Fish and chip shop	Bridge Street	Tommy Uttley
Fish and chip shop	Chapel Street	Livesey's
Ice-cream shop	Chapel Street	Jack Jessop
Sweet shop	Chapel Street	Fallow's
Cobblers	Chapel Street	Tom Oldham
Railway Hotel	School Lane	Unknown
Sweet shop	Birch Road	Waters
Hairdressers	Newsome Rd South	M Coldwell
Sweets and confectionary	Newsome Rd South	Stock's

The shops and businesses were all in addition to the eight Berry Brow Co-operative Society stores situated in Waingate. All those businesses in one relatively small village would take some believing today – but it was, and still is, a fact.

During the 1960s, every building in the plates section (figure 2) was demolished by Huddersfield Corporation (now Kirklees Council), in order to make way for new, modern, up-to-date housing. The residents of the village were re-housed in various areas of Huddersfield, much to the annoyance of many.

In 1955 my father's mother and father, who lived at 236 Meltham Road, Big Valley, Netherton, a couple of villages away from Berry Brow, bought a public house in Albert Street, Lockwood called The Star Inn. This became my early introduction to the licensed trade, in which I was to experience somewhat regularly in future years. Admittedly more at the customer's side of the bar rather than the proprietor's side, although I have spent a considerable time at that side over the years.

In the summer of 1959 they sold The Star and moved to Marsden, a village on the Manchester Road, approximately eight miles outside of Huddersfield, buying the Old New Inn, that was considerably larger than The Star. Unfortunately, my grandfather died in April 1963 after they had only been there for a relatively short time. Grandma kept the Old New Inn until her retirement in May 1971, moving to a house in Close Hill Lane, Newsome, some 300 yards from where we lived on Towngate. Shortly after Grandad passed away, my brothers Stephen and/or Glyn and I regularly helped Grandma at weekends by running the function room situated upstairs at the pub, whenever bookings had been accepted for various parties, etc. Yes – at that early age.

If the function was a late-night one, we would stay over at Grandma's, returning home the following morning on the Huddersfield–Marsden public transport. If it wasn't a late night, we would generally catch one of the later buses and return home that night.

I distinctly recall that on one occasion Glyn and I were waiting patiently at the bus stop in Huddersfield Town centre for the number 20 trolley bus that would take us back to Newsome where we lived. A car pulled up at the side of us, and the driver beckoned for us to jump in! Well – there was no way that would happen, as we had been brought up to be very sensible. Safety first had been drilled into us all – even in those days.

As it turned out the driver was Mr Clegg, who lived with his family just off Deadmanstone Road at the rear of the Co-op. With it being dark we hadn't recognised him at all. The very next morning he called in to see Mum and Dad to congratulate them for bringing us up as they had done, and he apologised for perhaps making us feel a little uncomfortable the night before. We genuinely hadn't recognised him.

Chapter 2

The School Years

When I was five, I started school at Newsome Infant School situated in the next village. Each morning my mother would walk me to the bus stop some 400–500 yards away where we would catch a trolley bus, an electrically operated vehicle which had two poles from the roof of the bus attached to overhead electric supply cables. The school was situated about a mile away, three bus stops, in Towngate opposite the top of St John's Avenue, Newsome.

I don't remember much about this school but do recall an incident concerning a Mrs Richardson. I can't remember whether she was a teacher or not but she certainly assisted during the school dinner times. On one occasion I clearly remember that prunes and custard were on the dessert menu. Not liking prunes (I still don't), I turned down the offer. Mrs Richardson did not like this and forced me to eat them, after which I was violently sick. That didn't go down well with her either. The following day, my mother took me to school as usual and gave her a very strong telling off.

I stayed at this school until I was seven and in September of 1956 started at Berry Brow Junior School, where Mrs

Richardson's husband was headmaster. In later years this school housed both infants and juniors. As it was situated between Birch Road and Caldercliffe Road, I didn't have far to walk to attend. It was totally different to the infant school and I enjoyed my time here much more. Everyone's favourite teacher here was Mr Halstead, and one could not wait to be in his class. In those days the teachers taught several subjects, so we all spent more time with our form teacher than with anyone else. Mr Halstead was famous at school (and had been for years) for the use of the large blackboard (it was in fact green) and a large wooden ruler. This ruler measuring approximately six inches wide by three feet in length was also used to "punish" pupils who had been naughty and deserved, in Mr Halstead's eyes, a crack on the backside with it. It was considered by everyone to be an honour, and I mean everyone, to receive this "punishment". Anyone who did not receive a whack was jealous of those who had and most of us did receive one (or more)! It was all taken in good spirit in those days, but I wonder how it would be viewed nowadays?

It was at this school that I became very keen on football during the winter months and cricket during the summer. It was the start of my sporting years. We played football in the schoolyard and occasionally during sports lessons at the 'Brow Rec. I became more and more interested in football and quite good at it. One year at this school, our classroom was being redecorated and the whole class was transferred to another village school, Stile Common Junior School, for a whole term. The headmaster was Mr Grout. He was, to say the least, extremely interested in sport and considered the school football team to be something special. I must have been considered quite a good player because I was immediately drafted into the side, playing right wing (number 7 – eat your heart out, Mr Beckham), the only pupil from Berry Brow to be invited to play for the side. I played all season for them –

even when we went back to Berry Brow School. Mr Grout, his Christian name was Wally, said that I was the best player to attend the school and play in the side since Ken Taylor, who played professionally for Huddersfield Town at football and for Yorkshire at cricket. Some compliment!

It was whilst living here that I had one or two incidents that caused me quite a bit of pain in more ways than one. I recall that at the time it was commonplace for some of the older kids, usually in their teens, to build wooden carts out of old pram wheels, timber, rope and other things. They were called lorry carts or sometimes soapboxes, and were quite fun to ride on and particularly drive – downhill, I might add. I was encouraged to have such a ride as a passenger on the back of a particularly fast one, built by a local teenager, Duncan Ward, who lived on Deadmanstone Road.

Partway down Chapel Street, which was the road immediately at the top of Waingate, and after reaching what seemed like a tremendous speed at the time, I decided that I wanted to get off. The driver wouldn't stop as he was having a speed test and thought he was Stirling Moss, so I threatened to jump off. Okay was the reply – so I did. Lots of crying, blood all over my clothes and the road, being carried home by a neighbour, a visit to the doctors, and three stitches across my eyebrow later, I decided that carts were not for me. My pain didn't end there, though.

My parents wanted to know whose cart I had been on. I lied and told them someone else's name, Rodney Haigh. When they found out the truth after confronting his mother, I had a pain elsewhere. Serves me right – but I didn't think that at the time.

Another incident happened during sledging in the snow at the 'Brow Rec. I was going downhill again (obviously) and failed to stop before I met the solid stonewall at the bottom of the slope. Oh dear, another couple of stitches from the doctor, this time in my upper lip.

Another one that springs to mind was on November 4th – mischief night! A few of us were going around houses, knocking on doors or ringing bells and then running away. This house's door was entered via the back garden as they had security lights at the front. The back was nice and dark – no danger here, we thought. Down to the back door we crept, hammered on the door and high-tailed it back up through their back garden. The big and very painful problem for me was that I had forgotten that their back garden was tiered and the very top of each tier was stone-flagged.

Yes – another trip to the doctors the following morning. This time no stitches involved. But guess what? It was the doctor's house that we were at the night before!

In 1960 I left the junior school and, having failed my eleven-plus exams, attended Newsome County Secondary School for the remainder of my school years, leaving at the age of fifteen at Easter in 1964. This school building had been a former mansion house owned by a prominent Huddersfield businessman and politician, Sir John Ramsden. It was situated in an area surrounded by woodland and adjoining the ever-popular Longley Park Golf Club. The access to the school from the village of Newsome was gained through an area called Squirrel Ditch. This area is to this day a much-sought-after area in which to live. Again, I excelled at most sports, including cross-country running, where I almost always came third in the annual sports day at this event. The winner was always Billy Meadows, who in those school days smoked like a chimney; second was always Philip Yates and third yours truly.

From a very young age, I have always been somewhat wary, even frightened, by water. I wouldn't even go paddling at the seaside without having my "wellies" on. At the senior school they had swimming lessons every week, and you can probably guess how I felt about this. My father decided to see the PE teacher, Colin Roberts, prior to me starting the school, about my problem. Dad knew Mr Roberts quite well, having been to the same school as each other and living in the same locality when they were youngsters. Mr Roberts told Dad not to worry about it and that I could attend the swimming lessons, sit at the side of the pool and only go in when I felt that I could do.

During the summer break prior to starting at Newsome School, a friend of mine, David Sykes, along with his father (Kenneth), suggested I go with them to the Cambridge Road swimming baths in Huddersfield and see how things went. I did so and, much to my surprise, I went into the water with them. Had my fear apparently been conquered? The new school year arrived, and Mr Roberts was ever so pleased that I would be able to learn how to swim. I was the last pupil in our school year to eventually gain my learner's certificate. Unbeknown to me at the time, whilst I was swimming the required length in order to be awarded the certificate, Mr Roberts had asked everyone to get out of the water, and when I had eventually completed the required length, they were all clapping and cheering at my achievement.

It was whilst at Newsome School that my time at the 'Brow Rec really started. I, along with my many friends of the time, spent many a happy hour playing football, cricket, tag, tin can squat, hide and seek, and many more games that were played at the time. There was very few television sets at home in those days, and computers, game consoles and the like were a thing of the distant future. We had to use our imagination as to what to do; electronics were not available in those days. But everyone always seemed to have a good time and enjoy the somewhat limited things that were available compared to those of today.

At the time, the football field was laid out adjacent to Ladyhouse Lane, the road leading from the village to the next village of Hall Bower. The football field today has been turned ninety degrees and one of the goal lines is now adjacent to the road. In those days the goal area closest to the fields was an absolute quagmire when it had been raining. To make matters worse for those partaking in the game, the quagmire was virtually 100% clay. When mixed with water it was like wearing lead football boots as opposed to leather ones. Your feet were virtually sucked into the ground, it was so sticky!

This is where I learned to play the game of football. Not so much with the school as with my friends of the time. As I improved my football ability, I was encouraged to play in the friendly matches arranged by the older children and teenagers. I considered this good for improvement. Some of the older players were extremely good ones and a few had trials with professional clubs from time to time, but, alas, without success.

A friend of my father had given him my first pair of football boots for me. They were made from the very hard leather of the day, were far from being supple and had extremely solid toecaps. The studs in the soles were made from leather and were literally nailed in place. If the leather studs became quite worn down in places, the nails obviously protruded and became a most dangerous piece of equipment. In order to keep these football boots somewhat "waterproof", a product called Dubbin was applied to them when they had dried out from the previous use. This made them very heavy to wear.

To make matters worse for everybody, professional footballers included, the actual footballs used in those days were also made of the same leather, had Dubbin applied to them and were even heavier than the boots we wore. Imagine trying to kick one or head one of these types of ball compared to the lightweight plastic-coated footballs of today. The players of today would struggle somewhat, especially when the pitch was affected by heavy rain and mud as it often was then. The pitches of the day were totally unprotected from the elements.

Around the time the school class were at the Stile Common School and I had been selected to play for their school football team, my father bought me a new pair of football boots. I was the envy of all. My new boots were no less than a pair of Stanley Matthews boots. Soft supple leather, screw-in plastic studs that were easily replaceable, no solid toecaps and more like shoes than anything I had seen before. Not only was I playing right wing, as did Stanley Matthews, but I had a pair of his boots!

Stephen and I made quite a lot of friends whilst we lived and schooled in Berry Brow, and I am very pleased to say that some remain friends today, although we live many miles apart from them now. My best friend at the time was undoubtedly Stuart Woodcock (Woody), who lived in Low Road, which was situated at the bottom of Waingate and across the main Huddersfield to Holmfirth Road, very close to the River Holme. In between Stuart's house and the river was a rookery, dozens of trees with rook's nests in them. We used to play in the rookery and by the river most days after school and at weekends.

A few years later, when I was working for Berry Brow Co-operative Society, the River Holme flooded, causing the rookery and farmland opposite to become completely submerged under the deep and fast-flowing waters. The road across the stone-built bridge spanning the river near the textile mill of John Brooks in Armitage Bridge, was closed to traffic because of the danger of it collapsing. The wooden pedestrian bridge across the river by the church was swept away and the river was flooded almost all the way into Huddersfield, some four or five miles away. (Figures 14, 15 and 16)

Some of my other friends at the time were David Armitage (Midge), David Crabtree, Michael Crabtree, Carol Clegg, Madeleine Clegg, Elizabeth Hicks, Judith Hicks, Alan Bates, Bobby Bates, Peter Boyes, Rodney Higginbottom and a few others whose names escape me – please forgive me?

I also became a member of Berry Brow Methodist Youth Club when I was around age fourteen. Walter Hobson and Brenda Walshaw ran the club, with help from quite a few others, such as Norman Taylor, Howard and Gillian Robinson, and Michael Early. We had some fantastic times there, and although I was Church of England and not Methodist, I used to attend the chapel regularly on a Sunday evening and occasional Sunday mornings.

Other friends from Berry Brow Junior and Newsome Secondary Schools and the youth club are too many to mention, but a few of my really, good friends were John Parkinson (Parky – whose parents had the Golden Fleece Hotel in Berry Brow), David Lockwood (Dilly), Philip Spencer, Robert Jagger, Alan Kitching, David Sykes, David Quarmby and Tony Morrison.

It was around this time that the youth club, with the blessing of the chapel, decided to hold what was to become an annual summer carnival. It was to be held on the 'Brow Rec and would involve various stalls selling food, drinks, bric-a-brac, lucky dips, etc., small sporting events, fancy-dress competitions and all sorts of things.

Another event was to be a pram race, whereby two people would form a team and race a pram around a pre-set course. Naturally there had to be a catch or two involved; it was not to be a straightforward, run-as-hard-as-you-can event. A good friend, David Lockwood, suggested that he and I have a go. We managed to find a suitable vehicle (pram) and duly entered for the race.

Race night arrived, and we were given instructions in respect of the course to follow along with the "catch or two". We were to start at the same time as the other teams and follow the course exactly or we would be disqualified. The catches were that one person would ride in the pram whilst the other person pushed the pram and load inside as fast as he or she could. At a given point the team had to change over, but not until each had drunk a quite large vessel of fizzy drink. Then it was away again as fast as you could to the next stopping point. Same again – change over driver and passenger, but not until both had drunk quite a large vessel of fizzy drink. Now, if you think that this should be quite easy for two fit young lads, you are quite right. But believe me, the quite large vessel of fizzy drink doesn't half leave its mark on you. There were another two or three stops and starts, yes, with change-over and fizzy drinks, but guess what? We won – hands down. The prize for winning, do I hear? A bottle of fizzy drinks each! But all enjoyed a good night.

A year or so later, I was to join the Berry Brow Methodist Pantomime Society, but more of this is to come shortly.

When I was fourteen years of age, we moved to the village of Newsome, as it had been decided by Huddersfield Corporation to demolish virtually the whole village of Berry Brow, in order to upgrade the village to modern standards of the time. This decision upset many of the villagers at the time and still does to this very day. There is a short film documentary on YouTube of the demolition, etc. – well worth a look!

We moved to No. 63 Towngate, Newsome, a three-bed council house, and guess what? It came complete with a bathroom and inside toilet! What luxury compared to the previous house. Now please don't get me wrong when I say this, as we had many a good family time in the house in Berry Brow, but the new house did have quite a few advantages in life.

I enjoyed my years at Newsome School, and although my academic achievements did not amount to much, I considered myself to have had a very good basic education. My thanks to all the teachers concerned.

Chapter 3

The Sporting Years

It really was in sport that I excelled. I became captain of the school football and cricket teams during my final year as well as being a prefect. Without doubt, the best and most successful footballer to attend Newsome School was Trevor Cherry. He was a year older than me and went on to play professional football for Huddersfield Town, Leeds United and England (twenty-seven full caps)! He also lived in the village of Newsome.

A year or two later, in the 1965–66 season, I was to experience first hand just how good he really was, as I was picked to play for the Huddersfield Junior Red Triangle League side in the Northern Area Cup Competition. We had practice matches against the likes of Huddersfield Town Juniors, in which team Trevor played at the time, and Barnsley Boys (the Barnsley AFC equivalent), in order to prepare ourselves as a team for the competition. It worked – we got to the final but unfortunately lost the match. I played in all the preliminary rounds and was also chosen to play in the final, but foolishly, although I didn't think so at the time, I declined the invitation, as I had also been invited by Yorkshire County Cricket Club to attend their winter nets for trials. This turned out to be a poor decision. I should have played in the football final – I now feel that I let the team and perhaps myself down.

When I was about twelve years old, I left Armitage Bridge Cricket Club where I had played as a junior and scored for the second team, and joined Hall Bower Cricket Club, where I remained playing until my retirement in the 1980s. With hindsight, I now believe that I retired too soon. However, hindsight must be a wonderful thing to have sooner than you eventually have it!

I started by playing with the junior under-seventeens and was soon encouraged to be scorer for the second team. Now in those days, if a side was short of a player or two in a game, through injuries or whatever, the scorer could bat, bowl and field for the side if he or she was registered for the club. Obviously were they doing all three they could not be scorer as well. In this case nearly all sides affected in this way would opt for their scorer to bat only and score for the remainder of the match. A substitute fielder would usually, but not always, be allowed and supplied by the opposing side.

This is basically the way that I started to learn the game and become reasonably good at it. I quite regularly batted when short of a player, but very rarely fielded, except of course when I was selected to play during holiday periods or when someone was unable to play at all for some other reason. I was of course appearing for the junior under-seventeens almost every week, even though I was much younger than most of the other players.

When I was fourteen, I was being selected to play almost every week in the second team and considered to be quite a good future prospect for the club. The following season, 1964, the second team captaincy was taken over by a player called Donald Higgins. Now, Donald was not considered to be of first team potential, but he was a schoolteacher by profession and he was a good leader and looked up to by the younger players. He was also a handy player and very rarely let the side down.

However, it was Donald that really gave me the opportunity to improve my game. I was a leading player in the Junior XI, but open-age cricket was something entirely different. I was a naturally good fielder, but Donald had spotted my potential for bowling in the Junior XI games, my batting as well, of course, and he duly gave me many opportunities to improve my game. I was very soon bowling and batting early in the innings and doing quite well on a regular basis. My fielding was, although I say it myself, more than impressive. Because of this I got the occasional game in the First XI under the captaincy and watchful eye of Tommy Galvin, at the time one of the best players and captains the club had ever produced.

The following season, 1965, I appeared in the First XI on the odd occasion again, mainly for my fielding, but wasn't good enough yet to command a regular place. I was still learning the game in the Second XI and Junior XI. That season the First XI were successful enough to reach the final of the Sykes Cup to be played at Fartown, the home of Huddersfield Cricket Club and at one time a fairly regularly used ground for county cricket matches played by Yorkshire. We were to play Meltham Cricket Club, one of the best sides in the league at the time, on a Sunday during August.

The selection committee duly met during the week to decide who would be playing in the final that Sunday, and it was decided that basically the same side that had represented the First XI for much of the season would play. It was also decided at the meeting, to appoint a twelfth man to act as a substitute fielder should the need arise due to injury, rather than rely on a substitute fielder from the opposing side. This decision was not one that was usually made. The twelfth man would also play should another team member be unable to play at all on the day.

Tommy Galvin, the captain, was adamant that only the best of fielders should be considered as twelfth man for the final. After some deliberation and a little arguing by one or two selectors, he got his way and Ian Graham was duly selected for the duty.

I understand that later a few players objected to my selection, as they believed they had more of a right than I had, particularly because they were older than me and had much more playing experience. I have absolutely no doubt myself, however, that I was, and remained so for many years, the best fielder at the club.

Unfortunately, Meltham beat us quite comfortably to win the coveted Sykes Cup.

The following season, 1966, I was very much a regular playing member of the First XI, and in the 1967 season we were good enough to be awarded the Byrom Shield as outright winners of Section A, the top division, of the Huddersfield & District Cricket League. The only other occasion on which the club has managed to win that trophy was in 1943, and, at the time of writing, has not won it since.

At this time each club in the league was allowed one professional player, who had to be registered with the league as that player. Should a professional become injured and unable to play, a substitute professional could be appointed. Most unfortunately this ruling was regularly abused, and quite a few clubs paid more than the one player allowed "under the counter" or "in their socks" to represent their club. I do not know of one club that would admit to this, perhaps even now all these years later, but I, and hundreds of others, knew that this was happening on a regular basis.

It was also in the early winter of 1966 that I was chosen to attend the winter nets by Yorkshire County Cricket Club for coaching under the watchful eye of one Arthur Mitchell, who was arguably the most famous of Yorkshire coaches ever.

I attended along with Graham Westoby of the Paddock Cricket Club. Never having been to the Headingley Cricket Ground before, we made our way by public transport, arriving well prior to the allotted time. We naturally made our way to the dressing rooms in order to change into our cricket gear ready for the session to follow.

Unfortunately for us, we entered the first team dressing room that was occupied by most of the first team players of the time. Even more unfortunately, they were not particularly happy to have a couple of young trialists in their dressing room and we were told in no uncertain terms to leave and make our way to the winter nets area situated underneath the stands. Needless to say – most of them didn't have much time for any of us during the day. The only exception being Geoffrey Boycott, whom, whilst we were padding up together, I found to be very helpful and informative, at least to me! Advice from such a source was very welcome indeed.

If I remember correctly, it was the winter that Geoffrey was trying to adapt from wearing spectacles to wearing contact lenses, and this was something we spoke about, as it is not really a good idea to wear spectacles in most sports at the best of times. Unfortunately, Graham and I were considered to be not quite good enough to be requested to continue the sessions throughout the winter.

In the 1971 season, we again managed to win through to the Sykes Cup Final, this time playing Elland, who were very much one of the best sides in the league. Unfortunately, we were beaten once again, as we were in 1965.

The following season, 1972, we once again won through to the Sykes Cup Final, for the third time in the club's history. This time our opponents were Honley Cricket Club, played once again at the Fartown Ground. After a very close encounter, we emerged as winners of the coveted Sykes Cup for the first (and only time at the time of writing) time in the history of Hall Bower Cricket Club. Our captain that day was Geoff Heywood, who had also played alongside two or three others, and me as twelfth man, back in 1965.

An interesting fact is that no fewer than seven of that cup-winning team came through the junior ranks at the Bower. Ian Booth, John Peaker, Barry Robertshaw, Geoff Heywood, Stuart and John Greaves, and myself.

It would be nice for the club if we could win it again soon – forty-nine years at the time of writing since our first and only success in the competition is a long time. The club did appear in the final of 1998 but once again lost to – yes – Elland!

Near the end of the 1972 season, a former Junior XI colleague, Peter Brook, came to watch a first team game at Hall Bower. He asked me if it would be possible to re-join the club the following season, and did I think he had a chance of making the first team.

When Peter had been playing in the Junior XI, he was a very promising fast bowler, and when I say promising, that is probably an understatement. We agreed that he would join the club the following season. It was then that Peter informed me that he and a friend, Bob Ainley, were going to climb the Matterhorn in February 1973. Most unfortunately both Peter and Bob were killed in an avalanche during the climb and his planned return to Hall Bower Cricket Club was not to be. The following is an extract that appeared in the *Alpine Journal* shortly after his death.

PETER BROOK 1947–73

> In recent years Peter had become a popular and well-liked climber, not only for his determination to climb difficult Alpine faces (his climbs need no review), but also for his understanding and love of people as portrayed in his songs and poems. His tragic death while descending the Matterhorn after making an impressive winter ascent with his close friend and regular Alpine companion, Bob Ainley, is indeed a sad loss to all of us who met

them either as friends and companions on some Alpine adventure or as humorous entertainers. As friends of both, I find it impossible to write of one without the other, particularly under present circumstances. Both were Yorkshiremen and extremely proud of it.

As a teacher in his home town of Huddersfield, Peter had gained a great deal of respect from 'his kids' as he called them. He often took parties to North Wales or Derbyshire, sacrificing his own weekends to introduce them to the mountains. As a young mountaineer he was outstanding: his stamina and courage, particularly in a tight situation, had to be seen to be believed. Had Peter not been swept down the Matterhorn by that totally unpredictable wind-swept avalanche he would have become in due course a truly great mountaineer. Perhaps his greatest virtues were his quest for fulfilment and his enthusiastic love of life.

Paul Braithwaite

(printed with permission of Alpine Journal)

In the 1977 season, Geoff Heywood, who was still captain of the First XI, asked me to consider playing mainly for the Second XI during that season, as he thought that my inclusion in the side would help them win the Paddock Shield, the Second XI equivalent of the Sykes Cup. I agreed to his suggestion and played mainly in the second team that season, only playing in the first team the maximum number of times allowed, therefore enabling me to also participate in the Paddock Shield competition.

My inclusion in the quest for the Paddock Shield must have helped because we reached the final, playing Thongsbridge Cricket Club at their ground, having previously been chosen by the league to hold the final there that year. Not only was I fortunate enough to be presented a winner's trophy along with my colleagues, but was also awarded the Cyril Laycock Trophy, as the man of the match, for an outstanding – yes, you have probably guessed it – fielding performance!

The Huddersfield & District Cricket League was, and is still, one of the top leagues in the north of England and, during my playing career, attracted some of the top players in the world to perform during the season. Some such players being Ken Shuttleworth (Lancashire and England), Alan Lamb (Northants and England), Dilip Doshi (India), Brijesh Patel (India), Madan Lal (India), Garth le Roux (South Africa) and others.

Prior to the commencement of my playing career, players of the calibre of Sir Garfield Sobers, Sonny Ramadhin and Wes Hall, all regular players of West Indies fame, also appeared and performed for clubs in the league.

Not long after leaving school, I joined Lockwood Civic Youth Club in order to play for the club's under-seventeens football team. A couple of my friends in the village also played for the team and it was they that suggested I also join to play for them. The team were trained by Les Clark, who also lived in Newsome at the time. The team were based in the Huddersfield Red Triangle League and played home matches at Moor End, council-owned pitches at the rear of the David Brown Gear Industries factory in Lockwood. We played almost every Saturday, and although we didn't manage to win anything, we became quite a good team. It was whilst playing for Lockwood CYC that in the 1965–66 season, I was chosen to represent the Red Triangle League side in the northern area cup competition mentioned previously.

It wasn't long before I was too old to play in the under-seventeens football league, and a few of my colleagues at Hall Bower Cricket Club were either playing for, or connected with, Newsome Working Men's Club football team. I was duly persuaded to join them, and I played here for a season before joining Berry Brow Methodist Football Club.

During the summer of 1967, Barry Bloy (see plates section figure 18), wrote to the manager of Halifax Town Football Club, Vic Metcalf, a former Huddersfield Town player, requesting a trial for himself along with "his mate Bill" – me, of course. I was working at the Co-op in Holmfirth at the time and didn't have access to a vehicle, so we travelled there by public transport. We arrived at the Shay football ground, the home of Halifax Town, at around 6.00pm, and met the trainer Clive, along with various members of the Halifax reserves team. We duly changed into our football gear and commenced training.

I didn't realise until we arrived that I knew two of the reserve team players very well but did not actually know that they played for Halifax reserves. One was the reserve team captain, Trevor Mallinson, who was courting Pauline Wilkinson, a member of the Berry Brow Pantomime Society. Trevor was a regular visitor to the rehearsals and performances, and I also knew his brother David, who had become a local referee after recovering from a broken leg whilst playing football in the Huddersfield League.

The other player was Stuart Greaves, who also played cricket for Hall Bower and had come up through the juniors there at the same time as I had. Stuart was a year older than I was, and I knew that he was a very good footballer as well as a cricketer but had no idea that he was playing with Halifax Town.

The first part of training was for all of us to run from the Shay to a local park a mile or so away in order to continue the evening's training. After various exercises were completed, we were split into two teams in order to play a game of touch and pass football. This is, of course, a normal game of football, but each player is only allowed to control the ball with their first touch of the ball and then pass it to a teammate with their second touch. If a player touches the ball consecutively for a third time, the ball is to be given up to the opposition and the game re-commences.

Now this way of playing was something I had been used to previously in training. Unfortunately, Barry hadn't played it before and was continually holding on to the ball and trying to dribble around the opposing players, therefore losing the team possession time after time. Barry and I were on opposite sides and he found it difficult and confusing to play this style of football. I suppose that I was a little fortunate as well, by being put into the same side as Trevor and Stuart – at least I knew two players names.

At the end of the session it was back to the Shay to change and go home. But not before I had somewhat of a couple of shocks. Following training, in which we had built up quite a sweat to say the least, we were instructed to take a cold shower prior to getting changed into our normal clothing. Wow – was that cold or was that cold!

The second shock was being asked to continue training with the team the following week at the same time. Unfortunately for Barry he was thanked for his attendance but informed that he was not quite up to the standard required. I later had to decline the offer, because as stated earlier, I did not have the means to get to Halifax from Holmfirth by the time required on the training evenings, as I did not normally finish work until 6.00pm.

During my earlier years of playing football at the 'Brow Rec, quite a few of the older players I referred to earlier were now playing for Berry Brow Meths, as they became known. I had only been playing for them for a very short time when Les Clark was appointed trainer at the club. Although I was playing at right wing when Les joined, he had other ideas, and I was immediately put into midfield. This was the position I was to remain in for most of my remaining football days.

We became a very good side in a very short space of time and had some really good players. Probably the best player we had was our team captain, David Early. David was a few years older than me and he also lived in Newsome. With me not having a car, he always offered me a lift to both home and away games. Huddersfield Town had been alerted to David's ability and a scout was sent to appraise him. Unfortunately, although the scout said that he was very impressed with his ability, he considered him to be a little too old to become a professional footballer. A lot of us thought not at the time, but at the end of the day he was still a 'Brow Meths player.

Around this time, quite a few professional players were studying and taking exams to be future trainers and managers themselves, after their playing careers were finished. A few professional clubs suggested that they obtain practical experience by training and coaching local league sides. One such player, I think it was Brian Hill, was asked to train the 'Brow. He did with a considerable amount of success, and the players appreciated it. Unfortunately, I was not one of them, as I was out with a long-term injury that took the best part of a year to recover from. I also missed a cup final due to this injury, as did David Early, who had received an injury during the semi final.

My injury had occurred at Hall Bower Cricket Club during the summer following my eighteenth birthday. I was assisting my father during an under-seventeens Walker Cup Final, who was looking after the ground at the time due to an illness suffered by Ronnie Wade, the club's official groundsman. I was foolishly carrying a bucket and brush in one hand, with a spade over my shoulder being held with my other hand. When I put the bucket and brush down on the grass, I let go of the spade that fell sharp end first onto my Achilles tendon, causing quite a nasty injury. I went to the doctors the following day, but he decided that stitches were not necessary. I then missed the rest of the cricket season and the whole of the following football season. I still feel that the doctor was wrong and that stitches should have been inserted.

The following season I rejoined Newsome WMC football club, where I remained playing until the mid 1970s, when I decided to call it a day. The heel injury was still causing me quite a lot of discomfort every time I played, even though it was well strapped up for every game that I played in. Unfortunately, I was never quite the same player again.

The regular Berry Brow team that I remember from those days was:

Wilson Rose

Stuart Ashton   John Tyas

Graham Turton   Alan Stafford   Geoff Ladbroke

Ian Graham   Ron Oddy   John Bray   David Early   David Oakes

Throughout the whole of my sporting life I was extensively supported, not only by my colleagues and teammates, but also by my parents. Particularly my father Kenneth (Ken), who was more than instrumental in my love of cricket and football. He was also involved at Hall Bower Cricket Club from my very early days and beyond. He was First XI scorer for many years, Junior XI coach for many years, looked after the cricket ground for a time and was also a committee member for most of them. He loved the club dearly.

My mother, Kathleen, not only made certain that the kit I was wearing was cleaned after every outing, but also ironed. She was a stickler for this and always said that if one can't make a clean and tidy appearance, one should not bother at all. She was also my doctor and nurse on the many occasions I returned home with an injury or two.

Thank you, Mum and Dad – I owe you both so much.

Chapter 4

Working Life Begins

A SHORT TIME before I left school, I went with my friend Bobby Bates to watch a pantomime performance at Berry Brow Methodist Chapel. I enjoyed it so much that I decided that I would join the Pantomime Society myself before their next production the following year. I had noticed a couple of girls in the production as well, of course! More of this to come.

I left school at Easter in 1964 at the age of fifteen and started work as an apprentice engineer at David Brown Gear Industries Ltd of Lockwood on the outskirts of Huddersfield. My father had arranged for me to start as an apprentice and he was also employed there as an inspector. He literally inspected finished items in order to ensure they were manufactured to the strict standards that the products and the company demanded. I commenced work at the David Brown Training School in the village of Scholes near Holmfirth, the last of the summer wine country, shortly after Easter.

Immediately prior to starting at the training school, I had been ill and commenced a week later than I should have done. When I arrived, the chargehand in the training department

I was assigned to informed me that I would have to share a workbench place with another apprentice, as all the workplaces had been allocated. The chargehand was called Philip Haigh and he was to become a good friend in later years. He was also promoted to Company Training Officer a few years later, a position he held for quite a long time. Most unfortunately, Philip is no longer with us, having passed away following an illness in the late 1980s.

The apprenticeship was based upon a course involving twelve weeks at Huddersfield Technical College studying for a Higher National Certificate in Engineering and six weeks at the training school. The other apprentices on the course were all a good year older than I was, and the majority had been educated at grammar schools or high schools, as opposed to a secondary school, as I had been. Consequently, they had learned more at school and were somewhat more advanced in various subjects compared to me. I was left behind in various subjects at college and the tutors didn't seem to care whether I was or not. Needless to say, I was not keen on the academic side of the apprenticeship, and although I was good at the practical side, I decided that it wasn't for me. After a few months I decided, against my father's wishes, to look for an alternative career.

My mother, who worked at Berry Brow Co-operative Society, suggested that I could do worse than apply for a job there. As it happened, a position shortly became vacant in the greengrocery department, which I applied for and was offered the position with an immediate start. Leonard Dickinson was the manager of the department and my mother had previously worked for him but was now in the drapery department.

She advised me that whilst Leonard's heart was in the right place, he could be, and quite often was, somewhat of a bully. Not physically, but mentally. Unfortunately, I was soon able to confirm that! Besides Leonard and I there was another departmental assistant called Mabel Horsfall, who worked almost full time. Mabel's husband was called Clifford and he was quite instrumental in my cricketing life at Hall Bower Cricket Club, being a former First XI player and Junior XI coach. Their son Geoffrey, who was three or four years older than me, was also at the cricket club for a time.

I had been assistant at the shop in Berry Brow for a couple of years when Frank Hartley, the driver of our mobile greengrocery shop, fell ill, and Leonard had to take it on himself to assume the responsibility of taking the unit out during Frank's illness. I very gratefully accepted the responsibility of stepping into Leonard's "shoes" as temporary shop manager. Not only looking after the daily running of the shops in Berry Brow and the neighbouring village of Netherton, but also in the ordering of additional daily stock when required, from the local wholesale market. To say that I revelled in the role would be an understatement!

It was whilst working here that I joined the Berry Brow Pantomime Society, as I had previously promised myself. In 1965 the annual production was to be *Cinderella* and I was invited to be in the chorus. Well, one had to start somewhere, I suppose! Rehearsals commenced, and I was enjoying myself, even though I could not sing very well at all. After a few rehearsals one of the principal actors, Stuart McLester, informed the producer, Constance Holmes, that he was unfortunately going to have to drop out of the production.

I had been showing a lot of interest in the production and had learned quite a few of the character's lines. When Constance asked me if I wanted to replace Stuart, who had been rehearsing for one of the comedy parts, I didn't need asking twice. I jumped at the opportunity. I enjoyed being part of the production tremendously, and the comments I received from quite a few of our customers at the Co-op encouraged me to continue with the productions over the next three years or so.

There was an occasion the following year that caused the script to be altered somewhat. I had to sing a short solo of a song called "All Together Now" during a scenery change. As I stated earlier, my singing voice leaves a lot to be desired. Anyway, onto the stage I went, and the pianist began to play the introduction notes for the song. I was absolutely petrified and started to sing so much out of tune that you wouldn't believe it.

On the spur of the moment, George Berry, who was playing the part of the usual pantomime dame, joined me on stage. He immediately stopped me singing and the pianist playing in our tracks and, in a loud and serious voice, asked what on earth was going on. I in turn stated that I couldn't help it if the pianist was playing out of tune and appeared to be tone deaf. Well, that brought more than a laugh from the audience. We then commenced to invite the audience to participate in the singing of the song – the women in the audience against the men. George invited all the ladies to sing together for the first verse and I invited the men in for the second verse.

Now all of this was totally unrehearsed, and it went down a treat to say the least – and all because I couldn't sing! This part of the show stayed in for the remainder of the performances and never failed to cause a tremendous laugh. We also took the shows to another Methodist Chapel in Brighouse each year and the reception to this part of the show was equally as good.

One year the pantomime was *Robin Hood*. Ian Whitehouse played the part of Robin, and in one scene had to shoot an arrow from his bow into a target off-stage. Naturally, the target was there for safety purposes. The moment came, and he duly fired the arrow with the deadly accuracy that one would expect of Robin Hood. Or so everybody supposed! The next moment the arrow came flying back onto the stage – he had missed the target by a mile and hit the wall instead. That caused one of the biggest laughs of the show – and not only for the audience.

In later years, Ian appeared on the TV game show *The Generation Game*, which was hosted by Bruce Forsyth, of course, and he won it! I wonder how that audience would have reacted had they been told about his accuracy with a bow and arrow? I have no doubts that Bruce would have played on it to the full!

I always played comedy characters and certainly had some good times in the shows, enjoying the company and friendship of the people involved in them tremendously.

Glenys Preston (now Smith) is still involved in various productions in the Huddersfield area and is a member of the Longwood Amateur Operatic Society that performs annually at the Lawrence Batley Theatre in the centre of Huddersfield. Another youth club member, Michael Hellawell, has also been very well known in operatic and acting circles in the Huddersfield area over the years, as has David Lockwood.

In 1967 Berry Brow Co-op was taken over by the Huddersfield Branch of the CRS (Co-operative Retail Services). The CRS greengrocery manager, who had responsibility for all the surrounding area branches, was called Alan Gray. He had previously been general manager at Mac Fisheries, a very well-known national company of the time.

Shortly after the takeover, the position of manager arose at a CRS branch at Hinchliffe Mill on the very outskirts of Holmfirth (*Last of the Summer Wine* fame). I was offered the position and gratefully accepted it. After a few months in the original existing greengrocery shop, it was decided to move the shop into a newer and much larger retail unit in Holmfirth itself, sharing it with the butchery department. The butchers was on one side of the shop and the greengrocery on the other. The manager of the butchers was Ken Littlewood, who was about the same age as my parents and lived on the same street, six houses away from us. Whilst Ken started work a lot earlier than I did, he always gave me a lift home after work.

I hadn't been working here long when I started taking driving lessons with a driving instructor based in Holmfirth, Geoff Brook. I don't remember how many lessons I had, but after a while the instructor suggested I apply for the driving test. I had the option of applying for the test at either the Huddersfield or Halifax test centres. The earliest test was available in Halifax and this was the option I chose. Not knowing the roads in Halifax, my instructor took me on lessons there for a couple of weeks for practice.

I managed to pass first time, although I thought that I was a little fortunate to, as I know that I made a couple of mistakes that I thought would cause me to fail. Obviously, the examiner must have considered the mistakes not too bad, or that I had coped with them satisfactorily.

It was some years later before I could afford my own car, but a few good friends let me drive or use their cars occasionally, including Ken Littlewood. In fact, Ken let me borrow his car a couple of days after passing my driving test, in order to have some stitches removed from my little finger, which I had cut quite badly the week before. It was very helpful, otherwise it would have been much longer public transport journey!

I was enjoying my time as manager in Holmfirth and was quite optimistic about my future. Unfortunately, in 1968, right out of the blue, it was decided by the hierarchy that late-night openings and all-day Saturday openings were to be introduced at several branches throughout the Huddersfield area, including Holmfirth. What a bombshell! What was going to happen to my sporting activities?

I requested a meeting with my departmental manager Alan Gray, in order to discuss the situation in more detail. At the meeting I was informed that the decision had been made and there would be no alteration. I was expected to adhere to the decision and work the different hours as required. After talking to my parents and thinking more about the situation, I informed Alan that I was not prepared to give up my sport and would therefore have to consider leaving. A day or so later I was informed by Alan, and the general manager of the CRS, a Mr Popplewell, that if I was not prepared to work the new hours, I could officially hand in my notice. This I did and commenced to work my notice.

A few days later I was offered the position as manager of a branch in another area of Huddersfield – Marsh – that was not being considered for the new opening hours. I declined the offer, stating that it would not be long before all the branches throughout the region would be expected to open in accordance with the new requirements. At the end of my notice period I was effectively without a job and reluctantly signed on at the Huddersfield Unemployment Office.

I had been unemployed for about six weeks when the grocery departmental manager at the Brockholes Branch of the CRS – Clifford Beaumont – contacted my mother, informing her of a vacancy at a company he knew quite well. He suggested that I contact them and request an interview, informing her that the company was an up-and-coming manufacturer of building materials and "going places". What an understatement that turned out to be!

The company was called The Hepworth Iron Company Ltd, a manufacturer of Vitrified Clayware Drainage Pipes & Fittings with various manufacturing plants throughout the UK. The head office and main manufacturing plant of the company was based in the village of Hazlehead, situated on the A616 between Huddersfield and Stocksbridge.

The position available was based in the sales office at Hazlehead, and after contacting the group sales administration manager, Raymond Hirst, I was invited to attend an interview the following day. I borrowed a friend's car and duly attended the interview as arranged. Raymond explained the requirements of the position and after a relatively short interview I was delighted to be offered the position. I gleefully accepted the offer and it was arranged for me to commence employment the following Monday. I was then introduced to my future colleagues and shown around the sales office complex.

The offices were situated some eight miles or so from where I lived, and Raymond suggested that I travel to work the following Monday by the Huddersfield to Sheffield bus service. He informed me of the time and where to catch the bus and that he would contact someone working at the company who would hopefully offer me a permanent lift to and from my new place of work. This was duly arranged with a Polish man called Charles Pukacz, who in the future was to become quite a good friend and colleague.

I commenced work on the Monday morning as planned and was welcomed to the sales office by the team manager, Malcolm Tomlinson, and allotted a chair and desk at my new place of work. My other sales office colleagues were Alan Penistone, Bob Lawrence, Robert Taylor, Keith Froggatt and Brian McCrea, who were all directly involved with the day-to-day telephone calls from customers, sales representatives and other area sales offices throughout the UK. Also situated in the sales office were Diane Carter, Carole Howard, Hazel Irving and Elizabeth Johnson, who were responsible for our entire typing and filing, etc. (Computers were a thing of the somewhat distant future.) The girls were joined shortly afterwards by Ann Buckley, whose father was one of the company's main haulage contractors, and Pat Farr.

Other employees that I had daily contact with were Geoff Dalton, John Hales, Dennis Schofield (who was also the professional at Broad Oak Cricket Club for several years), Stuart (Ned) Hodgkinson, Donald Moseley, Ira Mitchell, Neville Whitwam, Geoff Booth, Harry Manifold, Doug Shaw and many more.

Cupid must have been hard at work within Hepworth as well, as a few of the girls were to marry other Hepworth employees in the years to come. Hazel married Malcolm Tomlinson, Carole married Geoff Dalton, Ann married John Hales and I believe that Pat married Keith Crossland following a divorce from her previous husband, Derek Farr. Well done, Cupid?

My initial responsibilities were solely dealing with the issuing of credit notes and customer enquiries regarding any discrepancies or damages in deliveries made to them. Following a few days' training, I was virtually running my own small emporium and trusted to deal with the requirements of the job. I was also given sales brochures, price lists and catalogues in order to learn about the complete range of products manufactured and sold by the company. My new colleagues were also helping me to understand the requirements of the sales office, the products and were very helpful at all times. I was thankful to be accepted into the team without hesitation.

At the same time as I started my employment at Hepworth, another young man by the name of James Moorhouse also started. Jim, as he preferred to be called, had been appointed as an area sales representative and was undergoing product and company training for a few weeks prior to being released into his prospective sales area. The sales representative's immediate national manager was Ken Mansfield, who was also based at Hazlehead in an office immediately behind the sales office that I worked in. I am pleased, and indeed proud, to say, that both Ken and Jim were to become close colleagues and friends over the next twenty years or so.

Hepworth was basically a family company, the chairman of which was John F Booth. The managing director was a gentleman by the name of Peter Hinchliffe and his son Peter John Hinchliffe, was National Sales Director. Among other main executives at the time were Eric Crossland (Financial Director),

George Swift (General Sales Manager), Raymond Hirst (Group Sales Administration Manager) and Peter Brett (Conduit Sales Manager – Telecommunication Company Sales).

I enjoyed my introduction to the company via the "credit note" desk and found it very interesting learning the company's products through the reading and studying of the brochures and catalogues. My new colleagues were also very helpful in every respect, and it wasn't very long before I was encouraged to take a seat at one of the telephone sales desks. Another newcomer to the company, Peter Crossley, took over my previous position. I never looked back and revelled in my new-found career.

I found the job to be very rewarding from an actual working point of view, but unfortunately not from a salary point of view. The salaries paid by the company were reasonable, but not particularly competitive compared to, for example, builder's merchants employees, as I was to find out first hand in due course. However, the position and the actual job itself was, without doubt, the most interesting one that I have ever experienced throughout my working life. I took a real interest in everything that I did, worked hard and became quite successful in the environment.

I also started to become quite ambitious and decided that I would work as hard as I could and learn the products inside out in order to help me work my way up the ladder a little. Over the next couple of years, I developed a rapport with quite a lot of the customers, who were mainly builder's merchants, and some of them used to insist on waiting to talk to me rather than others who might be available immediately. The same could be said about the other members of the sales office staff, of course. They were all "top notch".

In 1970, not long after my twenty-first birthday, I bought my first motor car, a four-door, 1200cc Ford Cortina MK1 Saloon, maroon in colour. The registration number was JCX 950D and had originally been purchased from new in 1966 by Dennis Hill, who was an accountant and lived in Berry Brow. I knew Dennis from The Railway Hotel in Berry Brow, which was my favourite "watering hole". I paid the princely sum of £200 for it (the asking price) and sold it around eighteen months later for £140 following my move to Thomas Temperley & Son Ltd, as follows shortly.

After a couple of years or so, in 1971, I think it was, I applied to Ken Mansfield for a position as a sales representative that had become vacant in the area. Following several short discussions about it with Ken, he suggested that I wait a while longer and gain a little more experience before trying to take what he considered to be such a large step into the unknown. He was probably right in what he was thinking, and we became quite close colleagues. He gave me a lot of advice and help over the next few years, and I learned a lot from him.

I had an interesting time at Hazlehead and enjoyed my time working in the sales office tremendously. As I mentioned previously, my colleagues were second to none and we all got on with each other tremendously well. Everyone pulled together, particularly during extremely busy periods, and we all respected each other. I don't believe that I have ever worked with a better team than them – and I have worked with some very good ones over the years. The Hepworth Iron Company Ltd, along with all my colleagues will always remain in my mind.

Later in 1971 a local builder's merchants, Rock Mill Supplies Ltd, who were based in Sheffield, asked me to visit their premises one Saturday morning. They showed me around their depot and offered me a position as sales representative for them. After thinking about it over the next few days, I accepted their offer. They had offered me an increase in salary of £500 a year, along with a company car, complete with all expenses. It was too much for me to turn down and I reluctantly informed Raymond Hirst of the offer, and he in turn reluctantly accepted my notice, saying that he was not able to offer enough to deter me from leaving and that he would be very sorry to see me leave the company. I then effectively commenced my month's period of notice.

The following week, Raymond asked me to attend a meeting with himself and Peter John Hinchliffe. At the meeting I was informed that they did not want me to leave Hepworth and would I consider staying with the company if a suitable position should arise that I might be interested in. Of course, I said yes and added that I did not really want to leave, but the offer made had been so good that I felt I could not refuse it. Not only was the salary so much more, but the car and future job prospects appeared to be more in line with what I was aiming for. They then explained that a position had arisen at a company in Lancashire that Hepworth had very recently taken over.

Hepworth were at the time wanting to grow quickly and were very active in the taking over of competitors. I was offered a £500 increase in salary, a company car and expenses, along with the position of Sales Representative of Thomas Temperley & Son Ltd based in Bacup, Lancashire. Peter John explained that part of my brief was to bring the staff into the Hepworth way of thinking and working, especially in the passing of orders through to the most sensible Hepworth manufacturing plant, therefore maximising profitability for the group. I accepted the position and after a couple of weeks commenced working in Bacup.

The job entailed spending three days in the office taking telephone calls, etc. and two days out on the road making sales calls to various customers of the company. One of my new-found colleagues was Andrew Tomlin, who was also employed as a sales representative by the company, and his brief was identical to mine. Three days in the office and two days on the road. One of our joint responsibilities concerned driving to the bank in Bacup each Friday to collect the cash for the wage packets for all the employees to be made up. We had to inform the local police station as to the time we were collecting it each week, and they then arranged for us to be monitored whilst collecting it and driving back to the works a couple of miles away.

Things progressed quite quickly, but not in the way Peter John had briefed me and certainly not in the way I had expected either. Prior to Hepworth taking over, Thomas Temperley had been run as a family concern. The three directors were Hubert Tattersall (Managing Director), his brother, Fred (Works Director) and their father Horace (Director). The Company Secretary Edith Shepherd assisted them. Whilst Hubert remained the man in charge following the takeover, Fred and Horace remained a large part of the new set-up very much, as did Edith. None of them, Hubert included, took the slightest interest in adhering to the Hepworth philosophy of running the business in the interests of Hepworth. They continually ignored my repeated attempts to bring them and the company into the Hepworth way of thinking and working, as I had originally been briefed.

To cut the story short and to the point, it was I that was being indoctrinated into the Temperley way of thinking and doing things, and not the other way around! In a nutshell, they were simply not interested in changing their ways. It was not many months before I had had enough, and I made my feelings known to the Hepworth management.

During 1973, George Swift offered me the position of Sales Office Manager at Hepworth's offices in Bristol. Having had more than enough of life in Bacup, I accepted the position offered and duly commenced my new appointment with high hopes. After six weeks in the job, George informed me that I would be losing the company car that I had enjoyed with the job in Bacup, as it was not considered to be required as part of my new position. He offered me the princely sum of £6.00 per week as compensation. Now, even in the 1970s you didn't need a degree in mathematics to realise that you could not even run a car, never mind purchase one as well, for £6.00 per week (less tax, of course). I was job hunting again.

Meanwhile, back at Hepworth it was business as usual in the growth of the company. They had recently taken over a manufacturer just outside of Huddersfield, The Cumberworth Brick & Tile Company Ltd. This was a very small company manufacturing drainage pipes and fittings, but of the original salt-glazed type of product which required sand and cement jointing. This type of product was very quickly becoming a thing of the past. Raymond Hirst suggested to me that it might be in my interests to consider transferring from Bristol to Cumberworth, take over as office manager there and await an opening with more prospects within the group in the not too distant future. This I did, and I was allowed to keep the £6.00 per week!

The main reason for Hepworth purchasing Cumberworth Brick was to use their facilities to trial the manufacture of large diameter drainage pipes and fittings. By doing so, the large-scale production at their existing plants would not be affected by the trials which would take some considerable time to perfect. Production engineers and staff were duly transferred from other plants and the trials began. Production of the old-style pipes and fittings continued but was scaled down considerably. There was, of course, quite a large amount of existing stock that required selling.

Machines that were capable of extruding pipes and fittings in diameters of 15" (375mm) and later 18" (450mm) were installed and the trials were underway. The works manager, David Myers, was already employed by Hepworth at the Hazlehead factory, and was considered to be the man capable of succeeding. This he did, but it did take a couple of years to do so. Following the successful conclusion of the trials, the large diameter production was transferred to a Hepworth-owned unit in the midlands, Thomas Wragg Ltd. Eventually, a 24" (600mm) diameter range of pipes and fittings was successfully introduced.

Whilst working at Cumberworth, another builder's merchant approached me, A W Lumb & Co Ltd, a privately owned company based in the small town of Ossett, which is situated on the outskirts of Wakefield in West Yorkshire. I had known A W Lumb & Co from my early years at Hepworth but did not really know just what a prominent business it was in West Yorkshire. It was soon to become even more prominent.

It was in April 1974 and whilst working in the office at Cumberworth that I received a telephone call from David Briggs, a director of A W Lumb & Co Ltd. He informed me that the company was looking for someone to take over the responsibility from him for the day-to-day running of their merchant depot yard in order to allow him to concentrate on the development of the company, along with his fellow directors. He invited me to attend an informal meeting in order to explain the idea in more detail, if I was interested. I informed him that I was, and we arranged a meeting to be held at the home of David Lumb, the owner's son, for a couple of nights later.

I attended the meeting at David's house, which was situated only a short drive from my parents' house and was introduced to David, also a director, and Malcolm Roberts, who was the financial director. They informed me of the growth of the company over the last few years and explained their plans for the future development over the next few years. I was informed that if I was interested in joining them, David Briggs would train me in the running of the depot building products yard. My eventual responsibilities would include the control of the yard staff employees, vehicle drivers, stock levels and re-ordering, allocation of all deliveries made from the yard stock to the various vehicles on a daily basis. I would also be the first point of telephone contact in respect of all customer enquiries and for the placing of orders for all products purchased via the yard. I would also be the main contact for all drainage products manufactured by Hepworth.

It didn't take me any time at all to express my interest in the job in question to them, and they made me an instantaneous offer of employment. In addition to the eventual responsibilities of the position, I was offered a salary of £2,500.00 per annum (an increase of £750.00 over my Hepworth salary), a fully expensed company car (Ford Escort Estate), pension and health insurance schemes, and a fully expensed telephone installed at home. I quite naturally accepted their offer, which was made in writing the next day. I did have to inform them that I was required to give Hepworth three months' notice of termination of employment and was told that was no problem. I had also arranged to go on holiday for three weeks commencing late July and effectively commenced employment at A W Lumb & Co Ltd on Tuesday 14th August 1974.

I arrived at A W Lumb & Co Ltd early on my first day of employment some thirty minutes earlier than the normal starting time of 8.30am. I recall quite clearly that I entered the offices and awaited the arrival of David Briggs. A member of staff, Willie Raper, showed me into an office area and suggested that I wait there. I hadn't been there long when a man in what I considered to be in his sixties appeared. He had glasses on, was very smartly dressed and, whilst fairly small and of stocky build, certainly wasn't overweight. He asked me what I was waiting for and I replied that it was my first day at the company and I was waiting to see David Briggs. He introduced himself as Arthur Lumb and suggested that I wait with him whilst he went ahead and opened the company mail that Willie Raper had left for him. I was later informed that Mr Lumb always opened the mail each morning that he was at the office and that was the main thing he looked forward to most days. It was one of his ways of knowing what was going on.

I didn't have long to wait for David Briggs, and my first day of employment began by being introduced to my other colleagues. David Buddery – Director and Head of Concrete Product Sales, Barry Simpson – Concrete Product Sales Assistant, Pauline Bentley – Aggregate Sales Assistant, Pamela Harker – Secretary to the Directors, Margaret Burton – Receptionist, Liz ? – Secretary, David Lumb and Malcolm Roberts, whom I had already met, of course.

I was then introduced officially to Willie Raper – Trade Counter Clerk, and to the members of the yard staff – Steve Hudson, Phil and John Tomlinson. I was later introduced to the driving staff as they arrived back at the depot from their morning deliveries.

After spending a few days with David Briggs being shown the way the company and the yard operated, the pricing structures and various procedures that were required, it was suggested that I spend a few weeks at the trade counter, along with Willie, who would show me the way the yard currently operated. It was also a very good way to meet some of the customers that I would be dealing with upon a regular basis. Additionally, of course, I would be gaining knowledge in respect of the various building products that I had not previously experienced and, just as importantly, the pricing structures that were already in place.

I initially found it quite difficult working with Willie. He seemed to think that I was going to be some sort of a threat to him and was very reluctant to "educate" me in the terminology and the pricing of the products stocked and sold through the yard. An example of this was when a trade customer collecting products would come to the trade counter to book out products he required, or had perhaps already loaded onto his vehicle. Willie would deal with the paperwork which would require the product(s) and amount(s) collected and, of course, the customer's account number and name. Quite a few products had shortened terminology. For example, bags of cement would be referred to as OPC or SRC or Masonry. Customers would come in and ask me to book out, say, ten bags of OPC to them. When I asked Willie what OPC was, he told me just to write it down on the customer's collection note as that, and the accounts department would know exactly what to charge out on the invoice. It was quite a few days before I found out that OPC was Ordinary Portland Cement, SRC was Sulphate Resisting Cement and Masonry was Masonry Cement. It was the same with a lot of other products and I had to find out the hard way about many of them.

I was beginning to think that I had perhaps made a mistake in taking the job on and should have stayed at Hepworth. I had many a sleepless night worrying about the new job but was determined to win Willie over and succeed in it. After a few weeks it all started to come together, and I gradually came to terms with things, including Willie, who eventually became quite a good friend.

At the interview for the job I was offered a company car, but initially used my own car, an Austin 1300 Saloon, to commute from home to work and back. The company supplied me with access to their petrol account at garages in both Ossett and Huddersfield, and if I required petrol (or oil, etc.) all I had to do was drive in, fill up, give my registration number and sign for it. Very convenient – and I didn't have to pay for it either. I can't remember how much petrol was at the time, but when I bought my first car in 1970 it was four shillings and six pence per gallon. Today that equates to £0.225 per GALLON (4.5 litres) – work that one out at today's rates!

I had been in the new job for a couple of months and had still not been given an indication as to when the company car would arrive. I decided that it was time to ask about it and approached David Briggs with the question. David told me that they had been waiting to be sure that I was going to stay with them before making the not inconsiderable purchase. Later that day Malcolm Roberts informed me that the car had been ordered and should be available for collection within the next couple of weeks. Two weeks later, Malcolm drove me to Polar Motor Company on the outskirts of Barnsley to collect it. As offered at the interview, I was now the driver of a white 1300cc Ford Escort Estate. That evening I drove my father to the company in order for him to drive my car back home. I sold the car a few days later for a small profit! No – the Austin, not the Escort! I felt that I was now learning how to buy and sell, as part of my new job included being able to wheel and deal in respect of both the buying and selling prices of (at least) some of the products we dealt in.

I soon learned quite a lot about the company, the products that we bought and sold, the customers we dealt with, the staff we employed and was given an amount of freedom to negotiate with our customers and help determine the way the company operated the depot.

One of the first things I strongly suggested was that all customers, both trade and private, should book in at the trade counter PRIOR to collecting any materials whatsoever and obtain a "collection note" listing the quantities and descriptions of the products they required on that particular visit. Up to this point, many of the trade customers would just drive in and collect whatever they came in for before attending the trade counter in order to book the products out. They would quite often collect their requirements without the yard staff even knowing they were there at all.

After a short while I became aware that the yard staff seemed to be away from the actual yard in which they were employed to be, seemingly more often than they were actually there. They were there to assist the customer to load, if not actually load the requirements of the customer for the customer. They were also there to offload our supplier's vehicles and to put the stock into the required areas of the stockyard – were they not? You might not perhaps believe this next bit, but it is perfectly true.

The depot was quite large in size and in addition to the offices there was an outside stocking area (stockyard) and two quite large warehouses (sheds) in which products that were susceptible to weather conditions were stored. These products would include items such as bags of cement, bags of plaster and plasterboards, anything that bad weather might render impossible to use. One day I was looking for a yard staff member and couldn't seem to find any of them, so commenced to search the yard area unsuccessfully and upon entering the first warehouse, still no one in sight. Hearing a voice from the second warehouse, I entered it from the top entrance to find one of the yard staff searching the pallet racking quite carefully. It transpired that the three of them were playing hide and seek!

Well, to say that I was not impressed is an understatement to say the least. I let them know in no uncertain terms what I thought of it and them. They didn't seem to care much but they knew that I knew what they had been up to and that I was not prepared to put up with it. For weeks afterwards, I spent time during the day walking around the depot to let them know I was there. I have never considered myself to be a "dictator" and I do strongly believe that the workplace should be a happy place to work, but at the end of the day (and the start of the day) we were all there to work and being paid for it at the same time. If stupid activities affect the business, the business fails, and if the business fails, people find themselves out of work. Business owners put up a lot more than money to start the business in the first place, as I will refer to in a later chapter.

December soon arrived and with it the Christmas period. At the beginning of the month I was somewhat astonished to find that A W Lumb & Co were compiling a list of customers to whom a bottle of Christmas spirit would be given as a thank you for orders received. By Christmas spirit of course, I mean a bottle of whisky or brandy or some other product. I had seen plenty of bottles of such things at my grandma's pubs or the pubs I frequented occasionally (okay – more than occasionally!), but never so many in the one place. The company also received a considerable number of bottles from our suppliers as well, and the directors distributed all to staff members – everyone received something. I don't know whether any of the other employees received a Christmas bonus from A W Lumb & Co or not, but I was given £50.00 in my hand – and I had only been there four months. This was a very welcome and wonderful complete surprise, which I proudly passed on to my mother. I always thought that the chicken that Hepworth gave employees at Christmas was generous.

I had only been at Lumb's for a couple of months when I plucked up the courage to ask Pam out for a drink one evening. To my pleasant surprise Pam accepted and I spent a very pleasant evening in her company. Pam lived on the outskirts of Almondbury, only a few minutes' drive from where I lived. In fact, I had to pass where she lived every day whilst going to and returning from work. A few nights later we also went to a dancehall/nightclub in Leeds. We seemed to get on quite well and I started to get my hopes up a bit. We had a few dances at the Lumb Christmas dinner at Exit 22, a smart venue just off the M62 motorway in Ripponden. A few days later I asked her to join me for Boxing Day lunch at my grandma's house and she accepted. However, on the morning her father rang me at home informing me that Pam was not feeling well and unfortunately would not be unable to join me. Thinking the worst, I went alone. A day or so later Pam asked if I would like to watch a Huddersfield Town football match that weekend and if so, she would arrange a match ticket for me, but we would be sitting a few seats away from each other as she already had her ticket. I said yes of course, and she drove me to and from the match.

Just after Christmas it was her birthday (I didn't know until the night) and she asked me to join her and a couple of her friends for a meal at her house. I didn't need asking twice as I was becoming quite attracted towards her. The night came, and the meal and company were excellent to say the least – home cooking as well.

Pam's friends had come by taxi, and when the time came for the evening to end, I offered to drive them home. It was about then that Pam told me that she was going to Australia for a few weeks the following day. I asked her if I could return to the house to spend more time with her after I had taken her friends home. Pam said yes, and we spent the next couple of hours talking about various things, including her forthcoming visit to Australia. She told me that a previous boyfriend had gone to live in Australia and that she would be visiting him whilst there. Thinking the worst, I asked her to ring me and let me know when she had returned, but that was virtually the last time we met. Very shortly following her return she started dating David Lumb and they married a few months later.

1975 had arrived and things seemed to go from strength to strength for the company, and, of course, myself. We were picking up trade from all over the area and getting busier and busier. Unfortunately, the yard staff did not seem very keen on the upturn in trade; they had always been somewhat work shy, but the drivers appeared to be more than happy enough. David Briggs decided to purchase a fourth HGV (sixteen-ton GVW) lorry and a first non-HGV (7.5-ton GVW) in order to meet the demand that the increased trade required. I was also moved from the trade counter area into an office that was created for me from a previous storeroom that was situated directly next to David Briggs's office. Direct communication was that bit more convenient and I didn't have to walk across the yard getting wet when it was raining. I did continue to survey the yard and warehouses personally, though. The one problem with my new office was not being able to actually view the yard from it, as it was overlooking the rear of the offices on one side and the very high wall of the main warehouse on the other. What could I view? The gap between the two, along with a few items of stock, of course!

During the summer of that year, David Buddery advertised for a secretary to join his team in the concrete sales department. The successful applicant was a sixteen-year-old called Heather Cannings who lived in Horbury, a small town situated a short distance from Ossett. I didn't know it at the time, obviously, but in the next few months my whole life was about to change and in 1978 we were to marry, but more about this later.

The main entrance to the offices was via a door situated at the front of the building, a short distance into the stockyard. Employees' cars were parked immediately at each side of the doorway, which led into the reception area. Another entrance was situated just inside the main warehouse (plaster shed) and was used extensively when people needed to visit the trade counter or yard staff needed to visit the offices. This entrance/exit was only available via my office, so anyone going either way had to walk through my office, which soon became a bit of a thoroughfare. Not that I minded much – I did have my own office. Effectively, an employee who did not have their own car or who might park on the roadside outside the depot more often than not entered via this second entrance and then through my office, particularly when raining, as it was closer than the main entrance.

The bonus, of course, was that Heather used this entrance/exit virtually every day. We were soon to become a couple, although we obviously didn't know it at the time. After a few weeks of seeing Heather every day and talking to her, I asked her out and she agreed. Now Heather was only sixteen and I was twenty-six, and I was uncertain as to how she or her parents would think about the age gap. Another thought was would she or her parents wonder whether I had been in any previous relationship, serious or otherwise.

Well, I had had girlfriends from being about fifteen but had never had a serious girlfriend, as throughout the whole of my teenage years and into my twenties sport and then my career had been my main objectives. In my mid to late teens I seriously thought and hoped that I might become a professional cricketer or footballer, consequently concentrating on those passions. I was naturally attracted to girls but never really had the confidence to let them know, as I was particularly afraid of being rejected.

Heather and I started to go out together fairly often, with the consent of her parents, and soon became a couple, although initially we did keep things quiet at work.

A few weeks before Christmas in 1975 I was asked by David Briggs and Malcolm Roberts if I, along with my girlfriend, would like to attend a function in Doncaster with them and their wives to represent the company. I told them that I would very much like to but that they might not be very pleased to know who my girlfriend was. I was relieved when David said that he thought that it might be Heather! We all consequently attended the function, again with her parents' consent, but I don't recall to this day what her mother and father might have thought or said about it at the time.

During 1977 and 1978 business was improving continuously and the company was going from strength to strength. I had been introducing (with consent) a few new working practices in the yard and these did not go down well with the yard staff. John left and was replaced, Steve and Phil were not at all happy, and in 1978 I decided that it was time to put forward a change into the running of the yard. I proposed the introduction of a full-time foreman along with a couple of extra yard staff members as trade was getting much busier. I also felt that the appointment of a foreman would be extremely beneficial to the company in both the short- and long-term operations of the depot. The foreman would be specifically directing each member of staff in the daily operation of the depot, ensuring that all yard staff members were completing their jobs efficiently and to the satisfaction of customers, delivery drivers and not least the company.

It was obvious that the appointment could not be made from within and would entail being made from outside. I approached David Briggs with the suggestion of appointing a former colleague of mine who was currently the foreman at the Hepworth works of Cumberworth Brick. I had heard from a reliable source that it had been decided by Hepworth to move the large diameter production from Cumberworth to a works in the midlands at a factory known as Thos Wragg & Sons Ltd. Yet another company that had fairly recently been taken over by Hepworth. The Cumberworth factory would apparently be closed when the transfer arrangements had been completed.

It was agreed that I approach my former colleague, Philip Whitwam, with a view to him joining us and to invite him for an interview. At the interview Philip was informed as to the requirements of the job and he was made aware of the shortcomings of some members of the yard staff. He was duly made an offer of employment, and after discussing the offer with his wife Dorothy, he agreed to join us following his period of notice with Hepworth.

The day he informed Hepworth of his intentions, his former manager, David Myers, rang me and complained quite strongly that I was poaching his best staff. My reply was that I had been reliably informed that the Cumberworth factory was soon to be closed, as stated above, and that no doubt Philip and other employees at the Cumberworth factory may soon be losing their jobs. David did not deny this and ended the call without further confrontation.

A couple of weeks later, Philip joined A W Lumb & Co Ltd as yard foreman and commenced his role with enthusiasm and was accepted by the yard staff members without apparent problem. Once again, the company continued to grow busier and things were going from strength to strength. Everyone appeared to be happy and working towards the end result – a stronger and healthier A W Lumb & Co Ltd.

In the early part of 1979, somewhat of a bombshell was about to explode.

One morning David Briggs, Malcolm Roberts and David Buddery asked Bruce Turner (Malcolm's assistant), Barry Simpson and me to join them for lunch at The Kaye Arms at Grange Moor, as they wanted to discuss something quite urgent and confidential with us. Prior to lunch we were duly and very quietly informed that things were not all they seemed to be within the company. They went on to tell us that they were shortly to be asked to resign from their positions as directors of the company. The three of us were convinced that they were joking with us, but they were being absolutely serious. They preferred not to divulge the actual circumstances of the situation except that it was something to do with differences of opinion between the three of them and Arthur and David Lumb. There were three other directors within the company, Phil Scurrah, Brian Ward and Frank Webb, who were apparently backing Arthur and David Lumb in whatever the situation was. Not really a surprise.

They informed us that within a few days the inevitable would happen and that there was no reason why the three of us should not be asked to replace them directly as managers of our relative departments, as we were more than capable of doing so. They also advised us not to divulge to anyone within the company what we had just been told and to keep our thoughts to ourselves regarding the situation.

A few days later it all happened more or less exactly as we had previously been told it would. Arthur and David Lumb asked the three of us to go to the boardroom, where we were officially informed that David Briggs, Malcolm Roberts and David Buddery were no longer employed by the company in any capacity whatsoever and would not be returning to the premises. We were asked to consider replacing the three of them as managers of our various departments and that there would be no appointment of replacement directors in the immediate future. It was arranged for David Lumb to meet with us individually in order to discuss our new roles, which would commence with immediate effect. All three of us accepted our new responsibilities without hesitation and business continued more or less as usual.

I enjoyed my new responsibilities enormously and the company continued to grow as it had previously. Within a couple of years, the yard sales office had grown from three of us to six, the yard staff employees from four to six, drivers and goods vehicles from four to six, and the company was busier than ever. The other departments also grew similarly, and the accounts department was about to become computerised. Things were once again on the up.

The company had also purchased premises in Tamworth, Staffordshire, and A W Lumb (midlands) Ltd was established. It was to be run by a former Hepworth Iron Company Ltd representative, John Cureton, who, along with Arthur and David Lumb, was appointed a director of the new company. A member of the Ossett staff, Kevin Chapple, was transferred there as Yard Foreman from the outset. John Cureton was also appointed director of the parent company a couple of years later.

In 1982 an employee informed me that a number of customers were regularly stealing materials from the yard, quite often with the knowledge of yard staff. I reported this to David Lumb and it was decided to employ a private detective to ascertain what was actually happening and by whom. After looking into this we appointed a retired police inspector who had set up a small agency in Leeds. After extensive undercover "enquiries" spread over about ten weeks, nothing whatsoever was found out and it was decided by David Lumb to terminate the surveillance forthwith. With the help of a friend I had actually placed a bugging device in the yard sales office during the investigation in the hope of finding something out. Alas, it was to no avail, even though I was able to listen in to what was being said in there. I have not to this day mentioned about this device to anyone until now. The friend who provided the device, Brent Taylor, most unfortunately passed away during the summer of 1996.

I still believe to this day that what I was told was perfectly true and there was an amount of stealing going on – but by whom or to what extent I have no idea.

I think that it was during 1982 that David Lumb and his wife Pam went on holiday to the Lake District for a week or so. My wife Heather and I also spent a week there at the same time, but not with them, of course. In fact, although we all knew we were in the same area, we never came across each other's paths. It was at the end of the week that something rather strange happened.

A few months earlier, David had changed his company car for a Jaguar XJS. In dark green, it looked the perfect sports car. Apparently, the car broke down in Windermere just as they were starting the return journey from their few days away. David decided to take the car to the Jaguar main dealer in Windermere and left the car on their forecourt to be repaired. However, he apparently decided that he did not want to wait for the car to be repaired and instead purchased another vehicle, a Mini, in which to return.

Heather and I returned home the same weekend obviously not knowing what had transpired in Windermere. On my return to work on the Monday morning, Mr Lumb explained to me what had happened and asked me to return to Windermere to collect the Jaguar in order to drive it back to the office. The garage owner had informed him that they could not find anything wrong with David's car, which appeared to be fine and perfectly drivable. I rang Heather and explained the situation, and we both travelled back up to Windermere in order to collect the car.

On arrival at the garage the owner informed me that David had been somewhat offhand with him and insisted that as the garage was a Jaguar main dealer and the car was under guarantee, it should be repaired by them and returned to Yorkshire at their expense. He went on to inform me that they could not find anything wrong with it and that it should be removed from their premises. He did, however, advise me to drive the car steadily, keeping an eye on various warning lights just in case something wrong did develop. Heather drove my car back and I drove the Jaguar, both at speeds of no more than 40mph. It must have appeared quite strange to other drivers to see the Jaguar travelling at such a steady pace along the motorway network back to Yorkshire. It certainly seemed strange to me.

Upon our return the car was taken to the supplier for inspection, but I understand nothing detrimental or serious was found. The Mini (HEC 88X) was given to a new employee, Steven Liles, who had joined us a week or two beforehand, so it didn't go to waste, so to speak.

This sort of behaviour by David was unfortunately to become a little more regular in the not too distant future.

In the summer of 1984 a number of events happened that changed quite a few lives of employees at the company. A few months earlier I had employed Philip Whitwam's brother Kenneth as assistant yard manager due to the quite dramatic increase in trade through the yard. An appointment I was to become to regret. Willie Raper and his family went on holiday to Germany (his wife was German), as they had done for the past few years. As usual the yard was extremely busy, even allowing for it being the summer holiday period.

One particular morning, Bruce Turner came into my office, closed the door and told me that he had something very concerning to talk to me about. Very quietly he informed me that Willie had had a heart attack whilst on holiday in Germany the previous day and had unfortunately passed away. If this wasn't bad enough, he continued to inform me that the police had been conducting extensive inquiries for the past "few weeks" into allegations by a member of staff that a large amount of embezzling had and was still going on within the yard involving a number of staff members along with customers. Bruce told me that Willie was suspected to be extensively involved and that due to his tragic death of the previous day the police had decided to close the net around all concerned.

Bruce then informed me that the amount involved was in the region of £100,000 over the last few months. I asked him why I had not been informed of the police involvement and inquiries and was told that it was because the inquiries made by the private detective a year or so previously, at my request, had come to nothing. To make matters worse, one of the main offenders was suspected to be Kenneth Whitwam, whom I had appointed only a few months earlier. I do not know to this day who the other offenders were or whether they were employees or customers. What I do know is that other than Willie Raper and Kenneth Whitwam, no other member of staff was named or dismissed due to their direct involvement to my knowledge.

One casualty of the situation was, unfortunately in my

view, the yard foreman Philip Whitwam, Kenneth's brother. I had felt it necessary to ask Philip the direct question as to whether he was involved in any way or not. His reply was that he wasn't involved in any way whatsoever. I then asked him if he either knew or perhaps even suspected that his brother may have been doing the things he had been accused of. Again, the answer was no. I then advised Philip that if he did know, that it would be best for him to inform David Lumb as such because it would come out eventually and things would be much worse then.

A couple of hours later he came back to see me and informed me that he had actually known that Kenneth was being dishonest and that he had tried to deter him without success. He then told me that he was going to see David Lumb about it immediately and inform him as such. He also said that he was going to do this himself, as he did not think it fair to burden me with the knowledge that he had confessed to knowing, as he knew that I was a "company man" and that he respected me for that.

David Lumb decided to dismiss Philip with immediate effect, even though I tried to plead on his behalf that he be given another chance, but to no avail.

A few hours after the above events Steve Hudson asked to see me in my office that evening after the offices had closed. At this meeting, at which only he and I were in attendance, he immediately told me in no uncertain terms that if he were to be involved in this police inquiry in any way whatsoever, he would inform anyone and everyone that I was having an affair with someone. I retorted that with him saying something even remotely like that, he MUST be involved without question and that anyone with nothing to hide would in no way respond in that manner. I also told him that I would be reporting this "conversation" to David Lumb the following morning, as I certainly had nothing to hide. He said that he wasn't kidding and left without another word.

Before I left my office, I wrote down everything I could remember about that meeting, saw David Lumb first thing the next morning, told him everything that had happened the night before and gave him the notes I had made. David called Hudson into his office and confronted him. I don't know what was said but Hudson was immediately suspended from his job and subsequently dismissed.

Hudson later took the company to an industrial tribunal, which took place in Leeds. Our solicitors Eaton Smith & Downey represented Lumb's and I was asked to appear as a witness but was requested to wait outside the courtroom until such time as it might be necessary to give evidence. It turned out that I was not required to give evidence and the court upheld the decision made by the company to dismiss Hudson after what seemed to me a very short hearing.

A few weeks later a police officer from South Yorkshire Constabulary in Sheffield visited the company asking to see David Lumb. Unfortunately, David was away ill at the time and I asked if I could be of assistance in David's absence. It turned out that he wanted to know as much as I could tell him about Steve Hudson's employment at the company as he was suspected of being involved in "something" being investigated by the South Yorkshire Force. I was not informed as to what it was, but he wanted to know everything that I knew about Hudson, including why he had been dismissed a few weeks earlier! As far as I know we never heard anything else regarding this inquiry.

It was shortly before this situation that David was spending more and more time away from the company without anyone apparently knowing so beforehand. It was not like David to be doing this sort of thing and was totally out of character. It transpired that he had been experiencing something of a breakdown and was taking medication prescribed by his doctor in order to alleviate and help cure the problem.

One of the unusual things that David did was to purchase a canal boat. David had also had his driving licence withdrawn due to the medication that he was taking and had commandeered the services of Steve Hudson to act as his chauffeur on a full-time basis. They were both consequently spending a considerable time on the houseboat, which was originally based and moored in the Selby area. They later steered it via the canal system to the Calder Grove area of Wakefield.

I recall that David and I had a number of meetings arranged with our largest supplier, Hepworth Iron Company Ltd, that had to be cancelled and re-arranged due to David not being "available" on the days of the meetings. On the day of the latest occasion, I had to contact Hepworth in order to cancel the appointment, as David was, once again, unavailable. Our appointment was with the Hepworth Sales & Marketing Director, Bob Anderson, and UK Sales Director, Ray Bass, and we were due to meet at the Hepworth Head Office at Hazlehead at lunchtime. I was told in no uncertain terms by Bob, whom I knew quite well, that if David was not able to attend, then I was expected to do so alone!

I duly left my office almost immediately and drove the twenty miles or so to attend the meeting, arriving a little later than originally planned.

On arrival at Hepworth I was requested by one of the receptionists, Phyllis, who was employed there during my employment at Hepworth some ten years previously, to go straight to Bob's office within the main sales office on the first floor. This is where I had spent the majority of my time whilst employed by Hepworth. Ray, by the way, was a sales representative during that time and we had regular telephone contact during the course of business.

Bob immediately informed me that he had become very annoyed by the constant cancellation of meetings due to David not being available and that he was not prepared to accept this situation any longer. He stated that he was seriously considering closing our account with immediate effect unless I could persuade him otherwise. Having to think very quickly, I decided that I should inform Bob and Ray, who was also there, exactly why David had been acting in a manner totally out of character.

I explained the fact that David was currently taking prescribed medication and was only spending a little time at work, which was obviously causing a few problems. I also informed them that David had spent some time in a hospital due to the ongoing situation but that he was responding in a positive way. I did not, however, mention the various "happenings" that had been going on for obvious reasons. After a fairly taut start to the meeting they accepted that there was a problem that was in the course of being resolved and understood that it could take some time to do so fully. They asked me to keep them in touch with regard to David's progress and assured me that the information would be kept within.

Following the meeting I returned to the office but whilst driving back, decided not to mention the context of the meeting to anyone, in particular Mr Lumb, whom I considered already had more than enough on his mind with regards to David's erratic behaviour and continual instability. David continued to take his medication, and although he seemed to be steadily responding, he was still causing concerns for his father, staff and I assume Pam, his wife, more than anyone. She must have been under a lot of pressure as they now had a child, Fiona, as well.

In the early part of 1985, I started thinking as to how it might be to have my own builder's merchants as opposed to working for someone else. The more I thought about it the more sense it seemed to make. Could I make a success of it? I decided to put the idea to Heather and she was all for it. Heather was expecting our first child in August of that year but that did not seem to put her off the possibility. After all, it was going to take some time to put the idea into any form of fruition. We discussed the way forward together and I suggested that we needed a partner or possibly two, as the type of business I had in mind was not exactly a one-man band, so to speak.

After thinking about who might be interested in joining us in the idea, I decided to put the possibility to Bruce Turner, the accounts manager at Lumb's. Bruce was very interested, and we discussed the possibilities in more detail. We were both of the opinion that a third partner should be involved and decided to contact Mervyn Greenwood, whom I had set on at Lumb's a few years earlier. Mervyn was a few years older than Bruce and me and had recently left Lumb's to take up a management position at Howarth Timber, another builder's merchants in the area.

We continued to talk with each other about everything and decided to look out for a business to purchase rather than set up from scratch. There was very little available during the year, but we were not in any rush as we all had good jobs with the companies that we were currently working for. One area that we were all keen on as somewhat of a priority was for our new company to concentrate the business on as many cash sales as possible, along with the credit sales that tradesmen throughout the industry enjoyed, of course. Bruce and I had worked for Lumb's for some time and had experienced the effects of slow payments, disputes and bankrupt companies, knowing full well that we could not afford to jump into that area with a newly started business. Mervyn had also experienced similar situations, but from the other side of the fence, as a major construction company that he had worked for a few years earlier had gone into liquidation in quite a big way.

In August 1985 Heather gave birth to our first child, a daughter whom we named Laura, and I will expand on this in another chapter.

Heather received many good wishes, cards and flowers, including ones from colleagues at Lumb's and also from David Lumb and his wife. David was still receiving treatment but seemed to be improving. I was very pleased that David had thought of Heather through the problems he was experiencing.

Bruce, Mervyn and I continued to discuss and plan things as best we could, but nothing had yet turned up in regard to a possible purchase. During the Christmas holiday, of which the building industry usually closed down for almost two weeks, I started thinking that perhaps my place was to stay at Lumb's rather than risking everything on a new business. My thoughts at this time were totally with Heather and now Laura. Would it be fair on them to risk everything? Would it be fair to be perhaps working six or seven days a week, ten to twelve hours a day? Lots of things went through my mind during the holiday, making me think twice and more about the idea. I was becoming concerned that we might fail and that I would let the both of them down in a big way.

I now had more important responsibilities to consider than I had ever had before.

I talked my concerns over with Heather and concluded that I should remain in my position at Lumb's, rather than take what would have been the biggest risk of my life so far. On return to work in early January 1986, I informed Bruce of my decision and the reasons why. He was very disappointed but said that he fully understood the reasons behind my decision. I then telephoned Mervyn to inform him of the decision and he also told me that he understood my reasoning. I informed them both that if they should require any help with their continued efforts to start their own business, not to hesitate to contact me.

Business at Lumb's continued as normal for the next few weeks, but immediately after the Easter holiday, something totally unexpected occurred. Mr Lumb rang me from his office requesting for me to see him, as he had something to discuss with me. On entering his office, he asked me when it was my turn to hand in my resignation! Yes, just like that. I asked him what he meant by the question and he told me that Bruce had resigned that morning, as had Steven Liles, and that they were starting up their own business in Bradford. He then informed me that he assumed that I would also be resigning in order to join them, as we were all pretty close colleagues.

I immediately informed him that I had no intention of either resigning or joining them in their new venture and that I had no idea that they were intending to resign that morning. However, I did also inform him that during the previous year I had been thinking about joining Bruce, and a former employee, Mervyn Greenwood, about the possibility of starting our own business but over the Christmas holiday had a complete change of mind and had backed out, leaving Bruce and Mervyn to their own desires. I also informed him of my reasons for doing so and that I considered my future to be with A W Lumb & Co Ltd. I also informed him that I had absolutely no idea that Steven Liles had been recruited to take my place – which I didn't – until he had informed me so that morning. That really was a genuine shock to me at the time.

He accepted what I had said and thanked me for deciding to remain with the company and said that I would not be disappointed in doing so. He went on to say that I would have a job there for life. A football club chairman's statement to his team manager did not cross my mind – but on reflection, perhaps should have done. Bruce and Steven left the company that morning.

David Lumb was away from the company during this time and was actually in a hospital in the Leeds area undergoing treatment for whatever his problem was. Apparently, Mr Lumb, and possibly some of the other directors of the company, had decided that it was in David's best interests to do so, as the problem seemed to be getting worse. David had been becoming quite "erratic" and had been causing friction within the business and I assume that perhaps his private life was being affected to some extent also.

I think that it was during May or June of that year that Mr Lumb became more and more upset and concerned about David's state of mind and health that he came to one of the biggest decisions that he had probably made in his life. He decided that he had had enough of everything, that David's health meant so much to him that he no longer wanted the company. It seemed to be because of the company that David was in the state that he was. I have very recently been informed that the reason for the three directors resigning in 1979 was due to exactly the above. David had been going through a similar state of mind during the late 1970s, causing problems and embarrassment to colleagues and others, which I had not been aware of at the time.

Mr Lumb called a meeting of the directors of the company and informed them that he had decided to let the company go due to the ongoing problems with David's health issues. The directors informed him that they would possibly be prepared to buy the business from him depending upon the costs of doing so. Mr Lumb agreed to the possibility of that very much, as opposed to a sale to quarters unknown. It was suggested that the managers within the company should also be invited to join the small consortium, of which I was one. I did not hesitate for even one second to say yes please. Discussions went on between the directors and Mr Lumb over the next few days and a gentleman's agreement was made with regards the price immediately prior to Mr Lumb going on a two-week holiday to the Canary Isles with his wife, Noreen.

To say that I was very pleased in being invited to be included in the consortium would have been an understatement. To think that only some six months previously I had given up the opportunity of something similar with Bruce and Mervyn and I was now possibly going to be a partner in one of the biggest builder's merchants in the north of England – wow. Unfortunately, my excitement was to be a little short lived.

Upon return from holiday, Mr Lumb announced that he had changed his mind and was not going to sell up after all. More so, he stated that his son David would be returning to work almost immediately and resuming his responsibilities as managing director of the businesses in both Ossett and Tamworth. I don't believe that any of us foresaw Mr Lumb making the reversal, as David's health was very much a concern to both him and the family, and had been for some time.

I personally took the decision quite badly and began to think of the consequences of David returning to the company in the state of mind that he had been in for a considerable amount of time. I was extremely concerned that he would once again behave in the ways he had been previously. Going absent, missing appointments, upsetting suppliers, spending company money unnecessarily. A former colleague and director of the company very recently referred to David as being "a loose cannon" during his time at the company. Apparently, this was the major reason for his and other resignations, in 1979.

I rather stupidly (I came to believe later) expressed my feelings to two other employees, John Cureton, who was a director at A W Lumb (midlands) Ltd, and David Tingle, the sales manager for the concrete and aggregates department at Ossett. They were both part of the proposed consortium referred to earlier. In what I considered to be a confidential conversation, I let it be known that I was very concerned that David would not be able to re-commence his duties in the state of mind and health that he was in, and had been in for a considerable length of time. I also stated that I was uncertain that I could continue to work with David in those circumstances. What a mistake that turned out to be.

A few days later Mr Lumb informed me that he had been told of a conversation I had had with "someone" which was of a major concern to him.

Now I had always got on with Mr Lumb very well. In the past I had driven him to and from various evening functions, occasionally picked up shopping for him and his wife on my way home from the office, been invited to their house along with my wife for Christmas drinks and many other things. A few months earlier, David had convinced his father that we should open up a new depot in Sheffield. Not a bad idea, as we were delivering a lot of building materials into the South Yorkshire area and it made sense to do so. A promising factory and outdoor storage area were identified, and I was invited to inspect it along with David and his father. It certainly appeared to be perfect for our requirements and we were all of the opinion that we should take the idea further.

On the way back to Ossett we were discussing the possibilities and I mentioned that we should only go ahead with it if we were absolutely certain that we had the finances to do it comfortably. Not being on the board of directors, I was totally unaware of the company financial resources but was told not to worry about that. A few days later Mr Lumb called me to his office and reminded me of my concerns over the financing of the venture. He asked me why I had appeared to be so concerned, to which I replied that if it were to put a large strain on the Ossett and Tamworth businesses, the cost implications of a totally new depot could well result in the losing of the whole lot. I also reminded him that we were experiencing a slight recession at the time as well. A week later he informed that the idea had been shelved for the foreseeable future and thanked me for my concern and frankness in the matter.

Following Mr Lumb informing me of my conversation with the "someone", he never spoke to me again, not even to say good morning when we met, nothing!

Three weeks after that, David, who had now returned to work, informed me that he would like to see me in his office urgently. At the time I had been working on purchasing a new HGV to replace one of our older vehicles. I asked him if he would to like to see my vehicle recommendation, but he said no – only me. A good friend of mine, Brent Taylor, who was the Builder's Merchant Sales Manager of IG Lintels Ltd, one of our largest suppliers, was also in my office. Brent excused himself and said that he would come back in when I returned. I duly went to David's office to find him sitting at his desk and Ted Crabtree, another director, sitting in front but to the left of it. I was asked to sit down and was immediately informed that I was being made redundant with immediate effect. Furthermore, I was to clear my personal belongings and vacate the premises upon leaving his office. When I asked why I was being made redundant, he purely said that my services were no longer required and that I would not require replacing.

Well, I obviously knew that the real reason was that either, or perhaps both, John Cureton or David Tingle, had told his father. I immediately told him that was what I thought it was about, and that he was too much of a coward to dismiss me and was taking the easy way out. I also asked him why I had not been consulted with regard to what had allegedly been said by the "someone". He said that he was not prepared to discuss the matter any further and the decision made was irreversible. He handed me a letter confirming that I was being made redundant and that I would be receiving three months' salary in lieu of notice, that I could maintain the use of my company car for the duration of the three months but could not use the company fuel credit accounts. I was also handed a letter containing a reference, which, although I say it myself, was good reading. Before leaving his office, I asked if I could at least clear my desk after normal closing time rather than immediately, as I did have some self-respect! Some of the language I used was not fitting to include in this passage, but I have no regrets in using it.

Upon my return to my office, Brent came back in and could see that I was extremely upset. Upset to the point of actually crying, in fact. He asked what was wrong, and I naturally told him what had just taken place. He stormed out of my office without saying anything to return about five minutes later. He then told me that he had informed David Lumb in no uncertain terms that if David expected Brent not to keep in touch with me either as a friend or a future customer, he was going to be very much mistaken. Just after Brent left my office, Ted Crabtree came in and apologised for what had taken place just a few minutes before. He went on to tell me that neither he nor the other directors, to his knowledge at least, had been made aware of what had just happened. He also informed me that he personally had not even been made aware of my alleged comments to either Cureton or Tingle. I am absolutely certain that it was one of the two of them, as I had not discussed it with anyone else. Both Cureton and Tingle had quite a lot to gain by me not being part of the company, and to this day I have no doubts that they were very "happy bunnies" following my departure.

Naturally, Heather was very upset and concerned at the news, but reassured me that I would soon find another job. We discussed whether or not I should seek an industrial tribunal concerning the issue, as we considered that there was no legal reason to make me redundant. Effectively, I felt that if the Lumb family considered that my alleged comments had been sufficient reason to be punished in any serious way, I should have been dismissed, and not been made redundant. The situation of 1979 concerning the three directors, Messrs Buddery, Briggs and Roberts, came very much to mind, as they had as many reasons to have doubts regarding David Lumb as did I.

I decided not to pursue the industrial tribunal route and accepted that they obviously considered my comments to be untenable as they apparently had been in 1979 as above. I also realised that if I returned to the industry, particularly with a manufacturer, which was a distinct possibility, I would very likely have contact once again with Lumb's. If I were to pursue the matter, whatever the outcome, it would make it virtually impossible to do so. At least it probably would from their point of view. In the not too distant future, my thoughts regarding this would become reality, although I obviously did not know so at the time.

Even though I was quite upset about what had taken place, I have never forgotten how much I had actually enjoyed working there for the twelve years of 1974–86. I had learned a lot about the merchant industry, many different products from many different manufacturers, met and dealt with many buyers from building and construction companies throughout the UK, and worked with some of the best colleagues you could wish to. Even though I felt that Arthur and David Lumb had treated me somewhat unfairly, I felt very sad when Arthur Lumb passed away in 1988 (b. 1911) and his son David in 2002 (b. 1951). I was informed some time ago that David passed away due to a brain tumour, which, if that was so, might have explained his problems during the 1970s and '80s. However in January 2018, after attending the funeral of my mother's sister, Muriel, I visited Pam, David's widow. Pam informed me that David had actually died due to having cancer. It was very nice to see her once again.

The next three months were spent at home looking for future employment and being a "house husband". It seemed like an age before I finally secured a management position with a builder's merchant based in Bradford, Sam Rhodes & Sons Ltd. A family of four, the Carter family, who resided in the Huddersfield area, owned the company. A fifth director was Stephen Murphy, who knew the trading area very well. This position arose due to a recommendation to them by Barry Simpson, the buyer at Totty Construction Ltd, a Bradford-based construction company that Lumb's had dealt with for quite a time. I had dealt with Barry for quite a few years and we came to respect each other as business associates very quickly. We conducted a lot of trade between our companies for many years. Unfortunately, Barry, who was about the same age as me, suffered a fatal heart attack a few years later.

I was offered the position of depot manager at their branch in Mirfield, a small town between Huddersfield and Leeds, in late November 1986. I suggested that I should perhaps commence employment in January 1987, as it was so close to the Christmas holiday, whereby the majority of the building industry closed for around two weeks. It was a fairly long break to take but was originally introduced due to that time of the year usually experiencing cold weather and not much building work actually taking place. From an employer's perspective it made sense for employees to take part of their annual holiday entitlement during winter, rather than at times when the weather was much kinder for building and construction work to be undertaken. It was also good from most employees' point of view, as it allowed time to be spent with their families at a very important time of year, particularly for their children. However, my new employers insisted that I start at the beginning of December 1986, but at their main depot in Bradford, where I could learn the ways that they conducted their business.

I therefore spent the month in Bradford learning the ins and outs of their ways of doing things, which were a little different from which I had been used to for the previous twelve years. The month went pretty quickly, January arrived and so did Mirfield. I hadn't been at the Mirfield depot for long when they informed me that my new company car, a Mitsubishi Colt, was ready to be collected from a main dealer in Huddersfield. Up to that point I had been using Heather's car every day, which was a little inconvenient for her.

It seemed very strange to be working at the Mirfield depot compared with my previous time at Lumb's. I had enjoyed my own office there for a long time and to be suddenly sitting at a desk with a few others in the same room, all talking at the same time? I definitely was not used to that. The premises had absolutely no heating at all. Early in January the weather turned really cold and as the snow began to fall heavily, we were all in for a shock. The snow soon settled to a depth of six inches or so, obviously causing problems. It was a good job that customers were few and far between, as the forklift truck could not cope with the depth of snow as the ground became more and more slippery as the snow was compacted. We could not get our cars into the depot due to the gradient at the entrance and we had no heating anywhere on the premises. Overnight, the temperature plummeted to well below zero and underfoot the conditions outside became treacherous. Inside was not much better, for as well as the distinct lack of heating, all of the water pipes were frozen solid, and we couldn't even make a hot drink, never mind use the toilet facilities properly. For the next few days we had to bring hot drinks with us from home in vacuum flasks.

I naturally contacted the powers that be in Bradford with regard to the lack of heating in the premises and was informed that if we wanted heating – what a stupid thing to say – we could collect a "space heater" along with a couple of gas bottles the next morning from there. One of my colleagues, Chris Pitt, who lived in Bradford, collected them the next morning. That heater was welcomed with open arms at the time but didn't warm the place up anywhere near sufficiently. For the next few days overcoats, gloves and scarves were the order of the day. After a few days at last the water pipes thawed out and freshly made hot drinks were back in popularity.

I had been given full authority to negotiate prices with customers as I felt fit, on all the products that were available. Chris Pitt, whilst spending some time in the yard helping to load materials onto customers' vehicles, was also learning the office and sales side of the business, and spent quite a lot of time with me in the office. We were quite quickly obtaining new business, mainly from my previous contacts, and trade was improving.

By mid January I had more than a few occasions to question the accounts department in Bradford over a number of irregularities on customers' invoices. The accounts department in Bradford dealt with the invoicing of all the sales generated by Mirfield. Every customer collecting products from Mirfield would be presented with a document. This would consist of either a cash sale invoice or if the customer had a credit account a collection note. In the case of the latter we would send a copy to Bradford each day (by Chris Pitt, not by post), with the agreed prices on the copy in order for an invoice to be raised at those prices. Whereby products were delivered by our suppliers direct to our customer, the supplier would invoice us at Mirfield and upon receipt of the invoice we would check that the prices(s), etc., were correct, mark on the invoice the price(s), etc., to be charged to the customer, and take the invoice to Bradford for the accounts department to raise the invoice accordingly.

The system should have worked without a problem and did on most items we sent through to the accounts department. Then I started to receive a few queries from customers, mainly customers I had dealt with at Lumb's, stating that they were being charged different prices to those agreed. This was happening fairly frequently, and whilst I was informed by the accounts department that a credit note would be sent to the customers, it kept happening, often to the same customers. I decided to go to Bradford and try to see what the problem was, as it was happening too frequently for my liking. When I arrived there, I was informed by the owners' daughter, who as well as running the accounts department was also a director of the company, that they occasionally charged customers more than the agreed price which was invariably paid, and the invoiced price was not queried. I stated emphatically that I did not and never had worked in that manner in the twelve years I had been at Lumb's. Her reply was that I now worked for them and not Lumb's.

That immediately invoked me to look for another job, and after discussing the situation with Heather I started thinking where to look next.

Prior to taking the job at Sam Rhodes, I had been informed that The Hepworth Iron Co Ltd were closing a number of their northern depots in favour of opening a new depot in the Wakefield/Leeds area and were looking for a new depot office manager. I had previously attended a meeting with Raymond Hirst in order to discuss the vacancy and was actually offered the job. Unfortunately, the wage structure was no better that it was in 1974 when I had left them to join Lumb's. I turned the job down. But now that I had decided to leave Sam Rhodes I contacted Raymond once again to be informed that if I wanted the job, it was mine. We arranged to meet in his office at Hepworth a few days later to discuss things in more detail. We did so, and whilst the salary was considerably lower than that paid by Sam Rhodes & Sons Ltd, I accepted the position there and then. Raymond did offer me a company car along with running expenses, etc., which did help in making my decision.

Towards the end of January 1987, I handed in my notice, much to the annoyance of the directors, who asked me to reconsider, but I told them no, along with why I had made that decision. Chris Pitts also expressed his disappointment in the decision and informed me that he had been looking forward to learning a lot about the merchant industry from me. I duly left without serving my notice period of one month. The company was dissolved in the 1990s. Stephen Murphy later formed his own builder's merchant company, S B Murphy Builders Merchants Ltd, operating out of the premises in Mirfield, would you believe?

This next stage of my career took me back to Hepworth, commencing employment on 26th January 1987 as office manager of their newly formed Wakefield/Leeds Depot, situated in the village of East Ardsley, which is near to Junction 41 of the M1 motorway. Prior to actually moving into the depot I spent a week or so familiarising myself with the systems that Hepworth operated. The products were no problem, as I had been dealing with them ever since my first spell with Hepworth, virtually on a daily basis. But the ordering and invoicing procedures were now computerised, whereas in the 1960s and '70s everything had been handwritten and/or typed in the old-fashioned and somewhat sadly missed way.

Hepworth had also become a PLC rather than a virtually family operated limited company. The Hinchliffe family ties had ended and their involvement within the company was no more. Hepworth now had a chief executive officer in overall charge by the name of Sinclair Thompson. The position once held by Peter John Hinchliffe, and more recently by Bob Anderson, was now held by Ron Bradley but with the title of UK Marketing Director. George Swift, Ken Mansfield, Peter Brett and quite a few more were no longer employed by the company, but Raymond Hirst and most of the sales office staff were still there. It was good to be reacquainted and working with them once again.

One of my first unfortunate tasks was to visit the depots in Blaydon, Newcastle upon Tyne and Darwen (Lancashire), in order to ascertain whether or not various office files should be transferred to my new office in Wakefield. These depots were in the process of being closed completely, and most unfortunately the employees, many of whom I had known from my previous time at Hepworth, faced redundancy. It was not a happy start to my new job and one that I could well have done without, but the people concerned appreciated that it was not my doing and we parted company as we had always been – good friendly colleagues.

My visit to Newcastle upon Tyne was in the company of the North Eastern Regional Sales Manager, Roger Barton. In addition to visiting the depot, we met a few customers whilst in the region and spent most of the time together. A month or so after we returned to Yorkshire, Roger handed in his resignation to Ray Bass, who was still sales director. Apparently, Roger had decided to join his father in his engineering business in the midlands, following a number of previous requests to do so. He hadn't mentioned this to me during our short visit to Newcastle and it came as quite a surprise both to me and others, who considered he was well settled at Hepworth. A number of current employees applied for the soon-to-be-vacant position, and although I had only been back at Hepworth for a couple of months, I decided to apply as well.

I didn't get the job, but Ray told me that he was pleased that I had applied for it and that I had been seriously considered for the position. Apparently, it was felt that with me only being back at Hepworth for a couple of months, it may have caused resentment from longer-serving applicants who, had I been given the position, would have been working for me. I could understand the reasoning but was very pleased that I had been seriously considered. I then concentrated fully on the job in hand.

In addition to managing the newly formed northern sales office in Wakefield, my responsibilities included attending and participating in the monthly sales meetings for both the north-western and the north-eastern sales forces. Each month separate meetings were held under the chairmanship of that particular area's sales manager. The various area sales representatives would meet, discussions would take place and sales plans, etc. concerning each area were considered and put to work. I was not there just to observe but to also have an input, as my office was responsible for the receipt and transferring of information between the sales representatives, the sales managers, manufacturing works and other sales forces where applicable. Many of the orders generated throughout the region were also placed with the Wakefield office and transferred to the appropriate manufacturing and delivery plants. Any customers requiring the collection of products that Hepworth manufactured were expected to collect them from the Wakefield Depot rather than the main manufacturing works at Hazlehead, as had previously been the case. I enjoyed the job and the responsibilities involved, but the salary was disappointing and not as much as I had become used to.

I had been back at Hepworth for only a few months when a representative from another company arrived asking to see me. His name was David Rose, whom I had met many times when I worked for Lumb's. At that time, David was the northern area representative for Brickhouse Dudley Ltd, a prominent manufacturer of manhole covers and frames. He left Brickhouse Dudley and moved to another manufacturer in the same industry, Selflock Ltd, a few months prior to my departure from Lumb's. It was good to see him again and he informed me that he no longer worked for Selflock Ltd and that a builder's merchant based in Bolton, Lancashire, called Cooper Clarke Group Ltd, now employed him. He was now their newly formed Yorkshire Division Sales Representative working from offices based in

Pontefract. He asked if I could show him around the offices and depot, as they were very likely to be using us quite extensively once they had become a little more established.

I started to show him the offices first, and when we reached a quiet and unoccupied area, he informed me that the real reason for his visit was to ask me if I would be interested in taking a job with them as the manager of a new depot to be opened soon in the region. They had not at this time identified suitable premises and that I would initially be working from the Pontefract offices, with all deliveries being made either direct from manufacturers or the Bolton depot in respect of smaller quantity orders. I asked if I could have a day or so to think about it, but that I was definitely interested.

After talking to Heather about it and obviously finding out more about Cooper Clarke Ltd, I informed David that I was interested in finding more about the position.

One of the people I spoke to about the job, but mainly about the Cooper Clarke Group, was Alec McMurray, the North West Regional Sales Manager for Hepworth, with whom I had been working closely with over the previous few months. Alec knew Cooper Clarke Group quite well, as they were a substantial Hepworth customer of quite a few years standing. He was of the definite opinion that it would be a mistake if I did not take things further by meeting with them concerning the requirements of the position. I duly contacted David and informed him that I would indeed like to take things further. A meeting was arranged for a few days later with Peter Clarke, the managing director and founder of the company, at their head office in Bolton, and we talked extensively about the job.

I would be employed as manager of the newly formed Yorkshire Division, working alongside David Rose at the offices in Pontefract. My initial responsibility would, along with David, be to increase the customer base and product sales substantially from those currently enjoyed. The chairman, Bob Ashby, who lived in Pontefract, was actively seeking suitable premises large enough to stock the full product range of building materials supplied throughout the region. In the meantime, David and I were to set up the Pontefract offices, employ a secretary and build up a portfolio of customers, with the Bolton depot supporting us with deliveries into the region being made from their extensive stockholding.

I was offered a salary well in excess of that enjoyed at Hepworth, a company car and full expenses, pension scheme membership after a qualifying period, and health insurance for family and myself. Needless to say, I accepted the position and duly, reluctantly, tendered my notice to Raymond Hirst. I must confess that it was with regret, as Raymond and I had always got on very well with each other, even during the fourteen years or so between my first employment with Hepworth and the stint I was about to terminate. At the same time that I was appointed as manager at the Wakefield depot, it was announced by Hepworth that Raymond would be retiring at the end of the year.

His eventual retirement coincided within a few days of my leaving to join Cooper Clarke. A few days prior to his actual retirement Raymond came to the Wakefield offices to say his last goodbyes to the depot and office staff as, along with other employees, we had contributed to a retirement present for which he thanked everyone. If I remember correctly, one of the retirement presents was a new greenhouse, for which he was particularly thankful, as he was a keen gardener. I believe that the company also presented him with the company car that he had enjoyed for the previous year. It did not have a personal registration number, but the last three letters of the registration plate were RVH – Raymond's initials! He was a truly well respected person by everyone that had the pleasure of knowing him.

A few days after he retired, he sent me a letter apologising for not giving me his best wishes in my new upcoming position with Cooper Clarke. That says a lot for the man I came to respect as a manager, colleague and friend.

Many years later, in 2014, in fact, after my family and I had been living and working in Tintagel for almost twenty years, I had the inclination to visit Raymond and his wife during a visit I was making to Huddersfield. I called unannounced at his home only to be informed by his wife Ruth that Raymond had passed away some years earlier. To say that I was shocked would be an understatement. I had no idea of this and it wasn't something I had even contemplated. I spent about an hour talking to his wife, during which most of the time, we were both upset and also happy at our remembrances of a truly good husband, father and friend.

Letters to me, from Raymond just prior to his retirement in 1987 and of January 2015 from his wife, will be treasured for the rest of my life and are a testament to the type of people they were and still are. The letter dated December 2014 from me to his wife is, I think, self-explanatory (figures 27-29).

After duly serving my notice with Hepworth, I eventually commenced employment at the Pontefract offices of the Yorkshire Division of Cooper Clarke Ltd. I spent my first few days with Peter Clarke at their head office in Farnworth, Bolton, learning the "ins and outs" of the Cooper Clarke sales policies and some of the specialised products that they dealt in that were exclusive to them only. They were somewhat different to the normal builder's merchant in that they actually supplied various building materials to other builder's merchants as well as the construction industry in general. This was something new to me, but following my introduction to the various products involved and the special prices that had been negotiated with the manufacturer of those products, I fully understood and appreciated the reasons how this could be achieved.

In addition to the specialised products only available to the group, they were also supplying general products to other builder's merchants as well. This was achieved in two ways. Special discounts arranged with the manufacturer and in many cases collection of the products from the manufacturer using outside transport, which in addition to a better than normal standard discount, a discount for collecting the product was also negotiated. The result being, of course, that many products could be offered to other merchants, virtually at manufacturers' prices, without affecting the profitability to Cooper Clarke Ltd. The system was well thought out and when put into practice worked extremely well for all parties concerned.

Following my few days induction in Bolton, David and I commenced the task of building up the trade of the Yorkshire Division from our offices based in Pontefract. The office comprised of a large open-plan office, which incorporated the reception area for visitors, and a second office, which we used for displaying the various specialised products that the group sold. It was quite spacious and comfortable and served as a good base from which to operate prior to obtaining a suitable property in which to trade from permanently. Bob Ashby was actively looking for the perfect property to purchase and it wasn't long before he was successful in doing so.

In the meantime, David and I continued to build up our customer base using the stocks held at Farnworth along with deliveries made direct from various manufacturers. We had also employed a secretary, Janet Stones, who dealt with all our typing (computers were very new) and was also receptionist. All three of us were soon, thankfully, very busy and seemed to be well on our way.

One day, totally unannounced, Bob Ashby came to the office and asked David and me to accompany him to the head office in Farnworth for a meeting with Peter Clarke. We left Janet in charge and accompanied Bob accordingly. En route, Bob informed us that we weren't just going for a chat or another look around, but that he had found suitable premises in which to form the Yorkshire division properly, and Peter and he needed to discuss the situation with us in more detail.

Upon arrival we accompanied Bob to Peter's office whereby we were informed that our new depot and offices would be situated in Leeds. The company was to be known as Cooper Clarke Group Ltd, Yorkshire Division, Pepper Road, Hunslet, Leeds. It was only about a mile from Junction 42 of the M1 motorway and was therefore very handy in respect of deliveries or collections to be made via the premises. Bob informed us that we would call there on the way back to Pontefract after our meeting in order for us to see the premises first-hand. We were then told that it was being proposed that both David and I would be appointed as regional directors of the division, which would effectively be a subsidiary company of Cooper Clarke Group Ltd. This news was a complete surprise to both of us, but a very welcome one to say the least.

A few months prior to this Bob had quizzed me quite a lot about both my time at A W Lumb & Co Ltd and the company in general. Naturally I told him everything that I knew, including David Lumb's apparent illness and that David's father Arthur had at one stage decided to sell the company to the directors and management due to David's predicament. Bob asked me if I thought that it might be possible that Arthur Lumb would consider selling the company to Cooper Clarke group. My answer was that I thought it doubtful but obviously possible due to David Lumb's continuing illness.

Totally unknown to me, Bob decided to contact Arthur Lumb regarding the possibility of doing so. I don't know the details of the approach at all, except that Bob told me that a few days after his conversation with Arthur Lumb, David Lumb rang him telling him that Lumb's was not for sale under any circumstances and that Bob, or anyone else from Cooper Clarke, should refrain from ringing or attempting to ring his father about it again. As I state above, I didn't know that Bob was going to make an approach, but for Cooper Clarke to have succeeded in their interest it would undoubtedly have been a very shrewd move – both for Cooper Clarke and, I hope, yours truly. If only?

The new premises consisted of a large outside storage area of around two acres, which had been used as a coal storage depot, and consequently the surface of virtually the whole area required concreting. This was something that was planned to be done in the not too distant future, but in the meantime, we would use the area for the storage of the various products we would be stocking and selling on a regular basis. The offices were also quite large, too large for our immediate or indeed fairly long-term plans. We soon decided to sub-let one wing, and Reliance Security Ltd moved into that section a few months after we did. There was also a small warehouse in which we stored products that could not be stored outdoors.

We required staff to be employed in the offices, the yard and, of course, drivers for the delivery vehicles. I decided to approach one of my previous colleagues, Philip Whitwam, with the prospect of joining us as yard foreman. At the time Philip was employed by Building Materials Barnsley Ltd and had been working there as yard foreman for a couple of years. He informed me that he was quite happy there and didn't really want to change jobs, particularly to somewhere that was much further to travel to. He asked me to consider his son, Philip Jnr, for the position, and following an interview with him I did so. We also employed two assistants for Jnr., along with two HGV drivers for the delivery vehicles we had inherited from our parent company at Farnworth. In addition to David, Janet and myself, we initially employed two further members of staff in the office.

It wasn't long before we had built up more trade than we could cope with staff-wise, and another HGV driver and further sales office staff were employed. We were soon operating a very busy depot and were dealing with some of the largest construction businesses in the area, as well as builder's merchants, of course. We employed some people that had been previously employed by other merchants in the area who specialised in various products. Enquiries for these products were generally directed to them, but all the sales office staff were knowledgeable about the majority of the products we dealt in. They were all introduced to the specialised products we bought and sold, and soon became conversant with our sales structures throughout.

Not all was plain sailing, however, as I was to discover occasionally, much to my disappointment. One member of staff, Mark Heslop, had been employed by Cawoods Building Materials Ltd, also based in Leeds, not far away from our Hunslet premises. One day I received a letter from the manager there complaining very strongly about Mark. The manager had apparently received a fax from "someone" calling him various names and using bad language in doing so. The fax did not contain the name of the writer, but it did contain the Cooper Clarke name in the fax letter heading! It transpired that Mark and the manager had been in "disagreement" over various things during his employment there, and Mark had let him know his feelings when he left their employment in order to join us. For obvious reasons I had to bring this to Mark's attention and establish the accuracy and content of the fax, as it was sent from our address.

Mark did not deny sending the fax or of stating the content therein. I informed him that it was not right to involve Cooper Clarke in any dispute or criticism that he or anyone else might have, against anyone or indeed the company. I insisted that he apologise to the manager at Cawoods in writing, and because of the content within the fax, etc., that he would be receiving a written warning as well as my initial verbal warning as to his future conduct whilst employed by Cooper Clarke Ltd. I understand that he did so, but I never did see a copy of the written apology. I did, of course, write to Cawoods myself accordingly.

Another disappointment was also regarding an ex-Cawoods employee, Gavin Walker, who lived in Sheffield but had also been previously employed by Cawoods in Leeds. The starting and finishing times within the office were staggered between the sales staff in order to be open a little longer. Some were employed between 8.30am–5.00pm and others between 9.00am–5.30pm. Gavin was initially in the former category. At the start of his employment he was regularly on time and occasionally even a few minutes early in arriving. After a while he started arriving later and later on a regular basis. I asked him why, as it was not fair on the other members of staff. He said that it was due to the traffic conditions en route. I suggested that he should leave home a little earlier in order to ensure a timely arrival. He would not agree to that, so I moved him to the later starting and finishing times. That resulted in exactly the same late arrival situation along with the same excuse. I eventually informed him that I would have to reduce his salary accordingly – that cured that!

I had also employed John Addy from Hepworth, to specialise in underground drainage sales, and he settled in well. At least, until Mark Heslop took a disliking to him for some reason. I never did find out why, but after John reluctantly brought it to my attention, I had to intervene in order to alleviate whatever the problem was. A further slight problem was concerning the yard staff's canteen area. I had occasion to walk in there during a lunchtime and was absolutely disgusted to find waste food stuff that had been fermenting for what appeared to be days and days in an open bin. They were not at all happy when I complained and pointed out that it was a blatant health hazard, and even more so when I reminded them that there was a large skip in the yard that was emptied each week. It didn't take much to deposit the waste there daily. I also pointed out that it was an open invitation to vermin, which was an even worse health hazard. They took the point.

We built the division up quite quickly, and in addition to David and me we eventually employed three HGV drivers, three yard staff, two accounts staff, two sales representatives and four sales office staff. We all considered that we were doing a good job and contributing to the Cooper Clarke group profits.

David was a regular supporter and season ticket holder of Leeds United Football Club, which was situated fairly close by. Peter Clarke, one of the founders of the business, was a staunch Manchester City supporter and regularly entertained customers and staff at Maine Road, City's home ground. David suggested to Peter that it could be beneficial to the Yorkshire division to have a similar arrangement at Leeds United. The following season we were the proud owners of an entertainment box in which we could invite up to eight guests to watch each home game. In addition to the Leeds United home games we had preferential opportunity to hire the box for Rugby League International matches that were held there throughout the season. We were lucky in this respect as Bob Ashby was also chairman of the Rugby League at the time. We used the box for every home game throughout the season but not for the RL matches. The cost of the box was shared with another business that Bob owned – Ashby Roofing Ltd.

During 1988 it was decided to float the company on the stock market. Cooper Clarke Group Ltd would become Cooper Clarke Group PLC. A number of employees who had been with the company for some time were allotted a number of free shares in the newly formed PLC. I was not one of them, only having joined a few months earlier, but was able to purchase shares at a discounted price, being an employee. I duly purchased shares to the value of £400. Over the next few months the shares went up and down, as they generally do, but I held on to them. I will continue with this part of the story a little later on.

In 1990 Bob retired as chairman of Cooper Clarke to be replaced by a Nicolas Jeffrey, who was also chairman of a furniture business in Sheffield amongst other positions. He had been chairman for only a few weeks when, totally unexpected by me or anyone else within the division, it was decided to close the division with immediate effect.

I was actually at home ill in bed, when my wife Heather brought the telephone to me informing me that Brent Taylor needed to speak to me urgently. Brent was the national merchant representative for IG Lintels Ltd, now one of our major suppliers. As you know, I had known Brent for many years, and in fact he and his wife Roslyn were godparents to our eldest daughter, Laura, and we were obviously also very good friends. I took the telephone from Heather and Brent asked if it was true that the Yorkshire division had been closed down or not. To say that this question was a bolt out of the blue was an understatement and I told Brent so. I obviously told him that I was unaware if indeed it was and would ring the office in order to find out what on earth was, if anything, going on.

I rang the office and Tracey, one of our accounts staff, answered my call. She informed me that she was unable to say anything, but Ken Bevan, one of the main board directors, was there at our depot and wanted to speak to me if and when I rang in. I immediately rang and informed him what I had been told and asked him what was going on. He confirmed that the division was being closed down with immediate effect and all members of staff were being made redundant with the exception of the two sales representatives and David Rose. I told him that I was driving over immediately to see him in person.

When I arrived there some thirty minutes later, the only member of staff left at the premises was Tracey. Everyone else, office staff, drivers and yard staff, had been informed of the decision and requested to leave the premises forthwith. Furthermore, a number of vehicles from Farnworth were already there, being loaded up with materials held in our stock for transfer to Farnworth. The decision had obviously been made at least a little earlier than that morning or even a day or two before. Bevan informed me that I was also being made redundant, that I would be given three months' salary in lieu of notice and that I could continue to use my company car for the duration of normal notice but without running expenses. On that note I was also requested to leave the premises.

I was out of a job again and had been made redundant for the second time in my career. And it hurt! But not only me – it hurt Heather just as much. It was perhaps as well that our daughters were too young to realise what had happened.

I held on to the shares for quite a while, but they continued to go up and down and then down and down. Eventually, a few years later, Peter Clarke decided to return the company back to his own control as a limited company. He started to buy back the issued shareholding from whoever would sell them to him – at a vastly reduced price, of course! He offered to buy the shareholding that I had and consequently offered me what I termed to be a derisory price. I refused to sell them to him for less than the £400 that I had originally invested, with him to pay the costs of doing so. He again offered the low price and again I said no. About a year later I received another letter from him informing me that if I did not agree to sell them to him at the price he offered, I would get nothing at all for them as they would become defunct. My reply to him, in writing, was that I would rather get nothing for them than let him buy them back at the derisory price he had time and again offered. In other words, if he wanted them badly enough, he knew the exact price he had to pay for them.

I have not heard anything further with regard to the shares to date and more than probably never will.

At the time of writing I understand that Cooper Clarke Group Ltd is no longer, and a different builder's merchant group completely, now operates the depots at Farnworth and Swinton. Whatever happened to the Yorkshire division property at Hunslet, I do not know.

Initially fearing the worst, being made redundant for a second time did not give me any great feelings about the situation at all. Even the knowledge of receiving three months' salary in lieu of notice didn't do me any favours at the time. Fortunately, I didn't have long at all to wait, as the "jungle drums" began to play within a few days of the closure.

I heard that an opportunity was available as representative for the north of England and North Wales for a company called Samson Lintels Ltd, a manufacturer of steel lintels based in Cwmbran, South Wales. The commercial manager there was Jon Hanks, who had previously worked for IG Lintels Ltd. Having dealt with IG for a number of years and knowing Jon from those times, I decided to call him at the Samson offices in order to explore the vacancy in more detail. After speaking to him and explaining my position, he informed me that he would discuss the possibility with the general manager, Michael Miles. Now I didn't realise that Michael was employed there, but I also knew him from my A W Lumb days. Selflock Ltd, a manufacturer of cast iron and ductile manhole covers and frames, had employed him as sales manager. David Rose had also worked for Michael at the time, and it was David that introduced us during the mid 1980s.

As promised, Jon spoke to Michael, and I was informed that I would be contacted by a PR company who was dealing with the vacancy. True to their word, I was contacted the following day and arrangements were made for me to attend a meeting at a Sheffield hotel later that week. Within the next twenty-four hours I was informed that the job was mine subject to accepting the terms of employment, which I did. The following Monday I was on my way by train to the Samson offices in Cwmbran for my induction process as Northern Area Sales Representative. I was met by Jon at the railway station and driven to their offices to be welcomed by Michael and other members of staff. I spent three days there being introduced to their ways of working, along with what was expected of me in my new role, and enjoyed every minute of it. I then left for home and my new responsibilities in my new company car, a Ford Sierra.

My main area of operation was to be along the M62 corridor from East Yorkshire and Lincolnshire through to Merseyside and the whole of North Wales, which covered quite a substantial area, along with some beautiful parts of the country in which to travel. The area was turning over around £120,000 of business each year when I started out, and my remit was to improve this steadily but substantially over the next few years. When I left Samson four years later, the turnover in my area was in excess of £650,000 annually. An increase in excess of 540% and not at cut price rates!

Samson Lintels had been a privately owned company but was now owned by the John Carr Group. One evening during my induction I was introduced to the John Carr, managing director from Bristol, who asked me what I intended to do to improve the area I had been designated. My initial plan, I told him, was to increase the number of merchant stockists throughout the area, thereby enabling the Samson Lintel to be readily available to the construction industry users. The product list prices were quite favourable to the end users, and the merchant discounts ensured that the product was a viable proposition for the merchants to stock. We at Samson would also become active with the end users on behalf of the merchants as and when required. Samson already had a service available for informing the builder(s) which lintels to use over which openings within a building, therefore ensuring that the correct loadings were adhered to. The builder would supply drawings of each house type they were planning to build, and Jon Hanks would calculate the loadings that the lintels were required to take over each opening. Jon would then provide the builder and merchant with a detailed list containing the exact lintel that was required over each opening in that particular house type. All the lintels supplied were also labelled with the lintel type and loading details.

Samson operated in various regions, with the sales force in addition to me comprising of Ben Williams (south and south-east), Steve Williams (Ben's son, South Wales and south-west), Hugh Lones (midlands) and of course Michael Miles, who was available throughout the country as and when required. Michael also spent time both in the office and out on the road with us, meeting our customers and assisting us as required. Jon Hanks was responsible for all the office activity and for the taking off of lintel requirements from drawings provided by the end users and architects, etc. The works manager, Phil (whose surname escapes me but shouldn't), was in charge of the manufacturing process, procurement of materials and the engineering staff.

The Samson Lintel was originally designed and marketed by Ben Williams' brother.

The range of lintels comprised of a "one piece" standard lintel along with a specially designed "Biform" lintel that was effectively in two pieces locked together at the top and separated by a rubber strip. The idea of the Biform Lintel was to enable the outer leaf to be manufactured from stainless steel and the inner leaf in galvanised steel, therefore enabling the outer leaf to be much more resilient to the adverse weather conditions appertaining in various areas of the country. Being manufactured in the two different steels, the price was obviously much lower than it would be by using stainless steel for both the outer and inner leaves, which was the way all the other lintel manufacturers offered their equivalent stainless-steel product. Effectively, the rubber strip protected the two steels from any chemical reaction that may occur between the different steels. This lintel was also manufactured in galvanised steel on both inner and outer leaves in various loadings.

I commenced my employment and, working from home, steadily built up a network of merchant stockists throughout the region. I hadn't been with the company very long when Michael Miles asked Hugh and me to attend a meeting in Cwmbran. At the meeting he informed Hugh that he was quite concerned about the lack of business in Hugh's area. He told him that unless business improved quickly and satisfactorily, he would have no alternative but to replace him. Obviously, Hugh was very upset by this, and I offered to try and help him in any way that I could. Back at our hotel that evening, we had a fairly long discussion and I told him how I was approaching prospective customers throughout my area. He seemed to take things on board and the following morning we resumed work in our respective areas.

Over the next few weeks things hadn't improved much in the midlands and Michael decided to replace Hugh. After a month or so, a new representative was employed to replace him by the name of Dennis Rigby. Dennis and I immediately got on with each other, and as I had with Hugh, offered to help him settle into his job in any way that I could. It wasn't very long at all that trade in the midlands began to improve as Dennis nurtured his "patch" methodically and successfully.

The Samson manufacturing facility and offices were situated in the Llantarnum Industrial Estate on the outskirts of Cwmbran and employed quite a few people from the area, mainly in the factory producing the end product. I think it was during November 1990 that Michael informed the sales staff in strict confidence that the production facility in Cwmbran would be closing down completely just after Christmas and that production was to be transferred in its entirety to premises in Gloucester owned by the John Carr Group. Michael informed us that the production workforce was not going to be informed of this decision until the New Year. We were all surprised at the news, but of course the decision was not part of our remit; it was entirely in the hands of the hierarchy within the John Carr Group.

I was of the very strong opinion that the staff being affected by the decision should be informed immediately, and I told Michael so. I considered it extremely unfair that many of the people who were likely to be made redundant would be spending money on the upcoming Christmas period that they would be unable to afford after losing their employment early in the New Year. I was informed that the decision had been made and was irreversible. Immediately following the Christmas break the bad news was broken to all and obviously did not go down well. Within a short time, the production machines and existing stocks were being transferred to the Gloucester premises. Other than Michael, Phil and Jon, I don't think anyone else from the Cwmbran staff joined the new facility in Gloucester. New production and office staff were duly employed, and Samson continued from the new facility.

Over the next few months business continued to improve satisfactorily, particularly in the north and midlands areas of the country, and in 1991 it was decided to show the products at the building exhibition that was held annually at the National Exhibition Centre in Birmingham in order to attract a more national clientele. An area was booked within Hall 5, the main hall for our type of product, and arrangements commenced in order to exhibit the range of Samson Lintels for the very first time. A range of lintels was specially manufactured to exhibit, new product literature compiled, a stand on which to exhibit the products and display the literature, etc. was designed and built.

It took a lot of planning, work and effort by us all in order to make it the successful showing it turned out to be.

Michael had planned the stand to be manned each day by me, Dennis, Ben and Steve, in addition to himself, of course, and Jon would remain in charge at the office in Gloucester. We were all requested to report to the NEC on the morning before the exhibition was due to commence in order to arrange everything ready for the next day.

Heather, my wife, drove me to the NEC and helped us to arrange the stand before driving back home.

Accommodation had been booked for us all at a hotel called Jonathan's, which was about a twenty-minute drive from the NEC. Dennis and I shared a twin-bedded room, and Ben and Steve another, with Michael in a room with his partner, Alison, who was also assisting with our customer refreshments, etc. The hotel was not like any hotel that I had stayed in previously. None of the rooms were numbered and they all had names instead. Now the rooms were not in any sort of alphabetical order and were spread over three floors with access on all floors via narrow passageways. To make matters a little more interesting for guests, the passageways were not straight with rooms easily found, but went off in various directions. Admittedly, a plan of the building was given to all guests, but it really did take some getting used to, I can assure you. We did occasionally miss our way whether it was going to or from our rooms to the restaurant, reception or wherever. I don't think any of us got used to it – but it was fun.

The exhibition was a resounding success for us and we gained a considerable amount of new trade from it in addition to national recognition from builder's merchants, house builders, local builders, councils, architects and, not least of all, other lintel manufacturers.

Among the visitors to our stand on one occasion was the founder of Keystone Lintels, an Ireland-based company, Sean Coyle. He took a definite interest in our standard RL lintel, and he and I had quite a long chat. Prior to him leaving the stand, Sean quietly informed me that he would like to offer me a position with Keystone. I told him that I had only been with Samson for a couple of years and that I was very happy there. He said that he understood my feelings, but if I ever changed my mind to give him a ring. I have often thought since then – what might have been?

Another visitor to the stand at the exhibition was the Catnic Lintels managing director Peter Morgan, who must have been very impressed by what he saw, as a few months later Samson were bought from the John Carr Group by Catnic and another chapter in the short life of Samson Lintels began.

A few days before the takeover by Catnic, Michael asked Dennis and me to assist the Gloucester-based staff in a stocktaking for the month end. Now we had never been asked to help doing this before but didn't think anything untoward. Perhaps I should have done. We attended as requested, assisted with the stocktaking, which took almost all day to complete, and were invited to have dinner at a restaurant in Gloucester city centre later that evening along with Steve, Ben and Jon. After we had ordered a round of drinks and they had been brought to our table, Michael proceeded to inform us that Samson was being sold to Catnic and the takeover would be completed the following day. He told us that various Catnic personnel would be arriving at the offices the following morning and asked us to be there by 9am. We continued with our evening, but Michael was a little reluctant to tell us much more other than that we would be continuing as normal and that we had a lot to look forward to in the future. I was a little perturbed by the news, as Heather and I had, earlier that week, agreed with a builder to commence with a quite substantial extension to our house in Wakefield. I rang her with the news immediately upon return to our hotel that night. We decided not to worry about it and wait to see what the Catnic hierarchy had to tell us the following morning. If the news was not so good, we could cancel the extension, as they weren't starting things until the following month.

It seemed a very long night, as my mind was thinking about all sorts of possibilities as to what might or might not happen.

The following morning, we all attended the office and met in the boardroom. It wasn't long before the Catnic contingent arrived, which consisted of the managing director, Peter Morgan, and the national sales manager, Geoff Hirons. Peter Morgan duly informed us that Catnic were now the owners of Samson Lintels and that we would be continuing with our business in exactly the same way that we had been previously. That there would be no changes in management, production facilities, the office staff or sales personnel, and if anything, staff levels should increase. He also informed us that he himself had been extremely impressed with the way we, the sales representatives, had been carrying out our work in the field. We hadn't been detrimental towards our competitor's products but had been complimentary if anything, pointing out to our prospective customers the apparent benefits of the Samson products compared to others in the marketplace. He also told us that he was very impressed with the way we had conducted ourselves at the recent building exhibition, having visited the stand on a number of occasions.

I had known Peter and Geoff for a number of years through my previous employment with both A W Lumb & Co and Cooper Clarke Group. I had always respected them and had no reason not to now. I had a chat with Geoff about our impending extension at home, and after asking him if he thought that we ought to delay it for a time, his reply was that we should go ahead with our plans immediately but to make the extension larger! We did go ahead but with the existing planned size.

The following day it was back to normal and business as usual.

The Catnic management did not interfere with the way that we continued our progress, but some of their representatives, who had always seemed to complain about Samson's growth rate, continued to do so. From our point of view that was not a bad thing, as by doing so, it suggested very strongly that we were succeeding in our remit.

We had been under the Catnic umbrella for only a few months when Michael Miles asked me to be available to take an important telephone call from him at 11.00am the following morning. I had appointments in and around Manchester that day and at the requested time, parked my car in an appropriate place, and awaited the call. Michael duly rang me and informed me that due to the recessionary conditions appertaining at the time, Catnic had decided to make some redundancies throughout the group. He went on to inform me that Samson were included in the cull and had to make one of the sales representatives redundant. My immediate thought was that with Michael ringing me first with the news that I was probably the one. I asked him almost immediately if I was to be made redundant, but his reply was that he could not operate my area of business from the office in Gloucester. That was a relief.

He then informed me that the redundancy to be made was to be either Ben or Steve Williams, and that he intended to leave the choice of which one of them to them personally. My immediate comment to Michael was that it was an extremely unfair way for the decision to be decided. I told him in no uncertain terms that there would be only one outcome in any

Died 29.3.92

Sporting giant who was a perfect gentleman

George Boothroyd dies

HUDDERSFIELD sport today mourned the death of Mr George Boothroyd, a prominent figure in cricket and football circles.

Gentleman George, as he was affectionately known, died in the Royal Infirmary yesterday afternoon after a short illness.

The 73-year-old was a real character who first made his mark as a professional cricketer in the Huddersfield League and as a goalkeeper with Huddersfield Town.

Mr Boothroyd, who lived at Waterloo, played football and cricket in tandem until just after the war when the summer game then held sway.

He was no mean achiever at cricket, developing into a fine all-rounder, and he was a professional for Shepley, Armitage Bridge, Broad Oak, Paddock and Kirkheaton as well as Bradford League club Spen Victoria.

Subsequently Mr Boothroyd played as an amateur for Brook Motors and was still playing after the age of 60.

Mr Boothroyd also became a respected administrator in both sports. He was a vice-president of the Huddersfield Cricket League, chairman of the Junior League and had helped organise Huddersfield's Joe Lumb Cup team for over 30 years. He also became

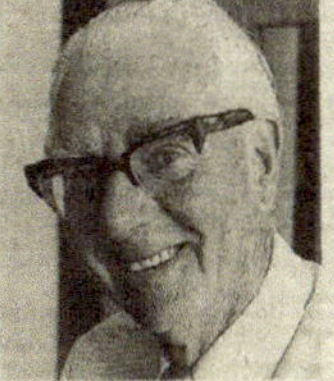

George Boothroyd — sporting ambassador

an umpire and was still officiating in the middle last season.

He was a keen follower of the fortunes of Yorkshire County Cricket Club and a regular attender at the Scarborough Festival.

On the soccer front Mr Boothroyd began a long association with the game at Berry Brow before making a Christmas debut for Town against Manchester City in 1940.

Mr Boothroyd later went on to play for Halifax Town and Bradford City as well as Frickley Colliery and Mossley.

Like cricket, his involvement in soccer did not end when his playing days were over. He continued to give his experience for the benefit of others and he took up refereeing and went on to complete over 40 years with the whistle. Always a distinctive and authoritative figure, he was instantly recognisable in his black beret.

Mr Boothroyd became a member of the Huddersfield FA in 1972 and was a vice-president, and he was also president of the Huddersfield Red Triangle League before it folded in 1984.

Mr Boothroyd was a true gentleman, always ready to quietly admonish any player or official whose behaviour fell below his own very high standards. He will be sadly missed by everybody connected with sport.

He was also a keen churchgoer and was for many years connected with Berry Brow Methodist Church and more recently Huddersfield Parish Church. Before his retirement Mr Boothroyd was a senior wages clerk at Brook Motors.

Mr Boothroyd leaves a widow, Winnie, and the funeral service will be at Huddersfield Parish Church on Thursday at 1.30pm, folowed by cremation at Huddersfield Crematorium.

Figure 1

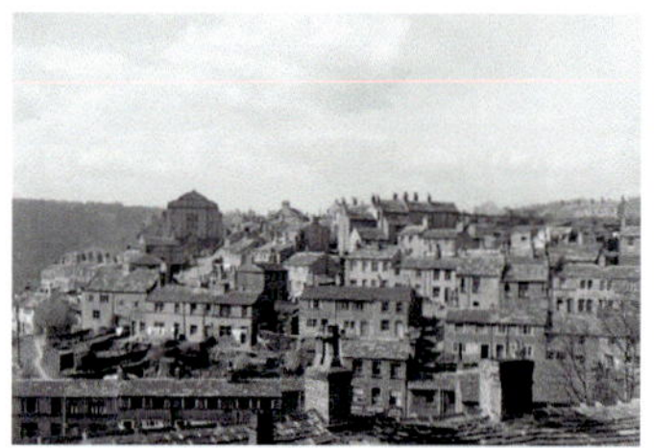

Figure 2

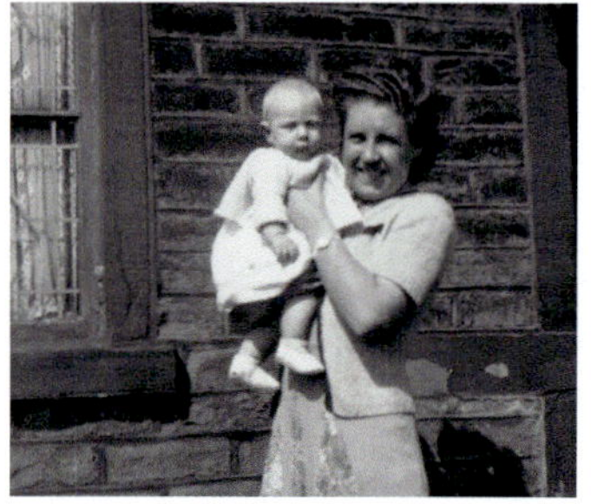

Figure 3

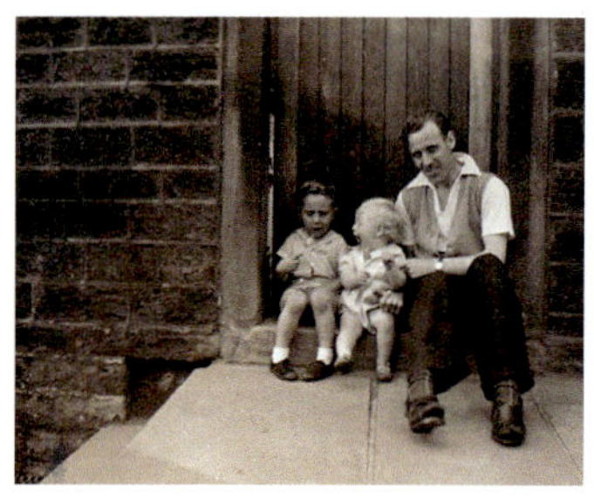

Figure 4

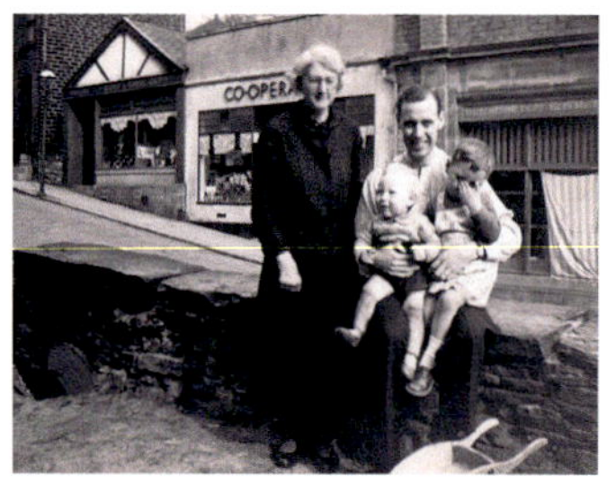

Figure 5

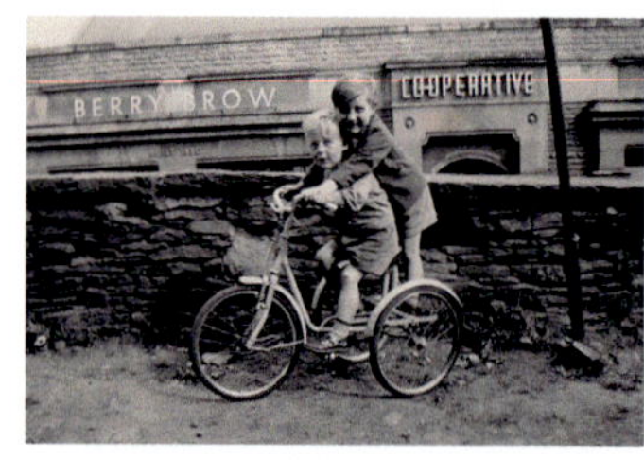

Figure 6

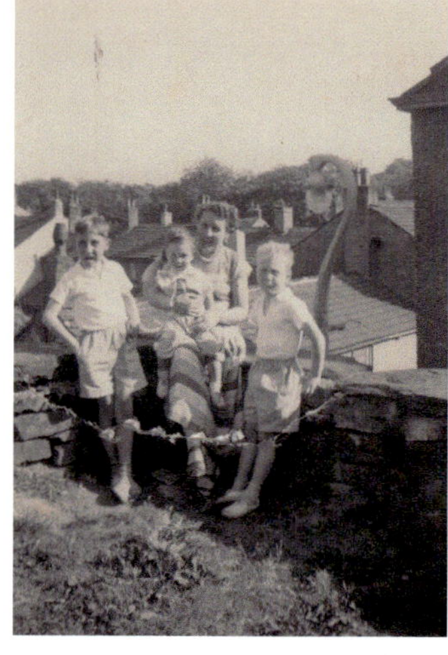

Figure 7

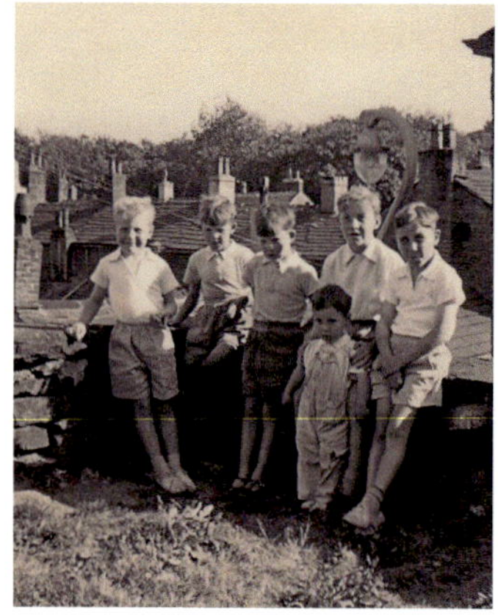

Figure 8

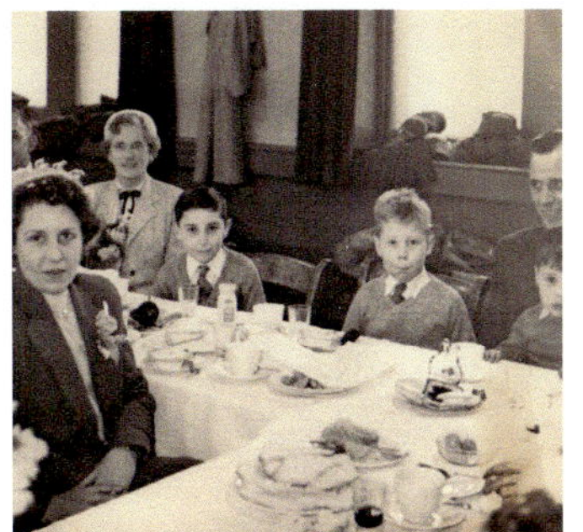

Figure 9

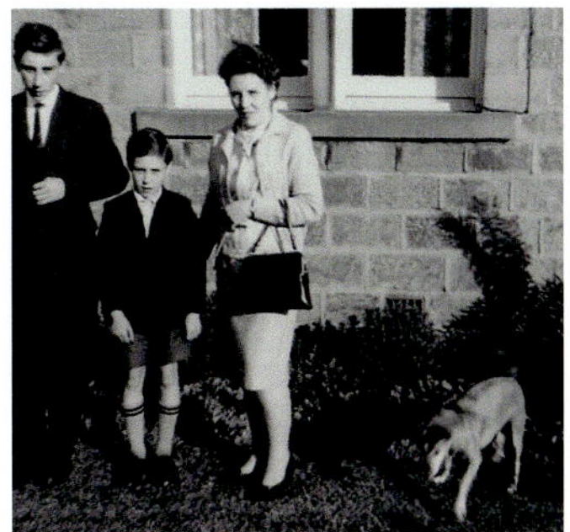

Figure 10

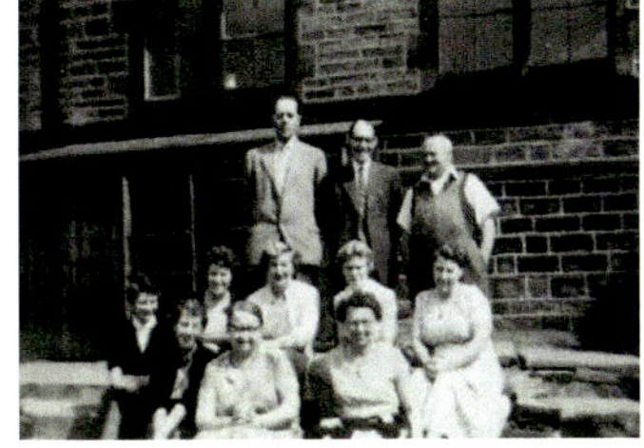

Figure 11

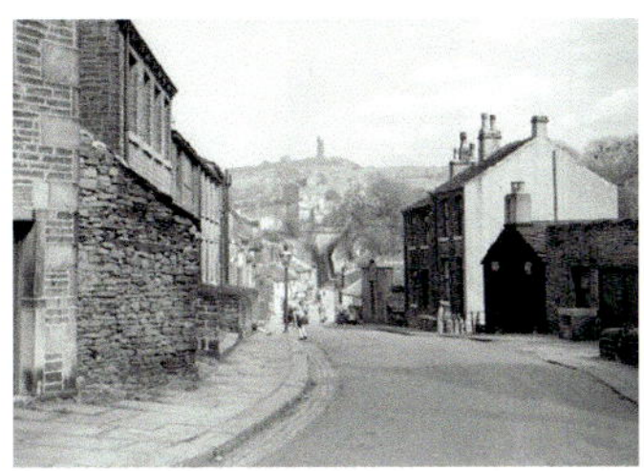

Figure 12

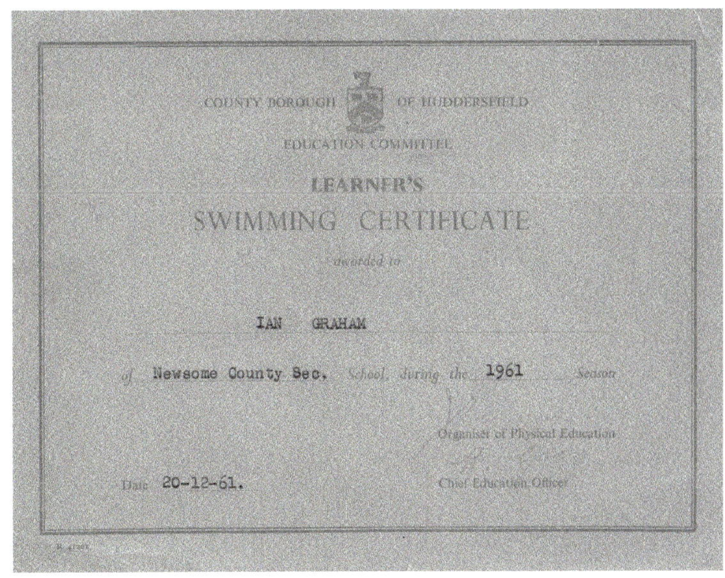

COUNTY BOROUGH OF HUDDERSFIELD

EDUCATION COMMITTEE

LEARNER'S

SWIMMING CERTIFICATE

awarded to

IAN GRAHAM

of Newsome County Sec. *School, during the* 1961 *Season*

Organiser of Physical Education

Date 20-12-61.

Chief Education Officer

Figure 13

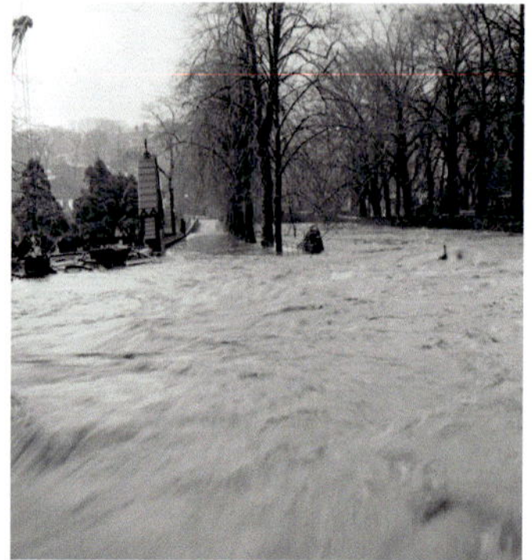

Figure 14

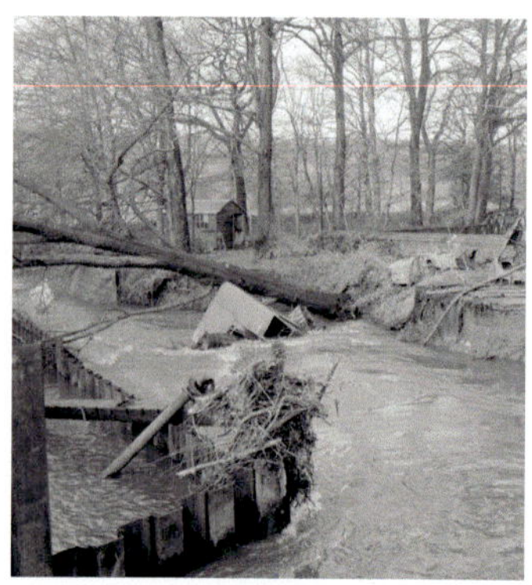

Figure 15

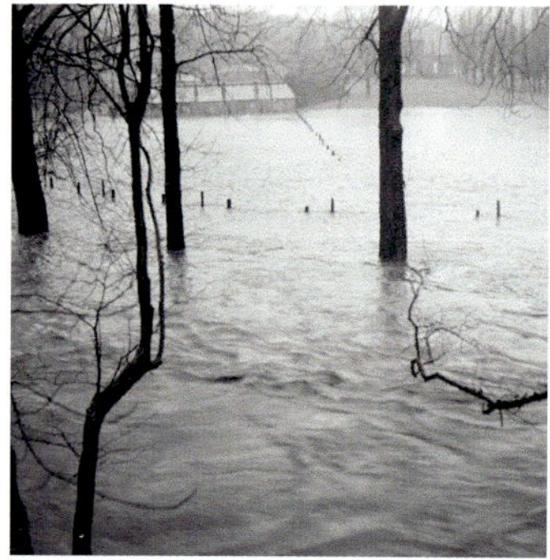

Figure 16

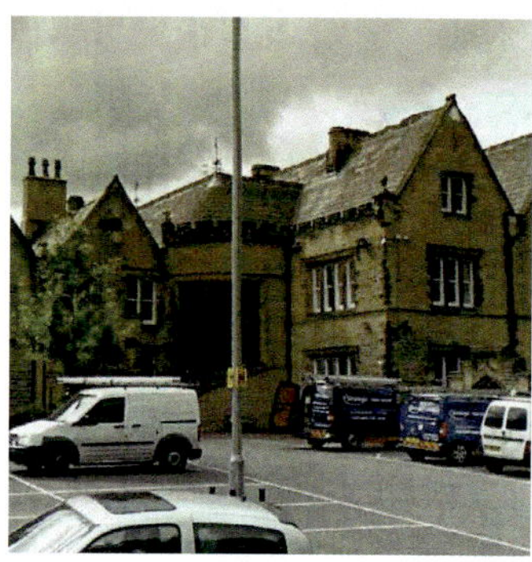

Figure 17

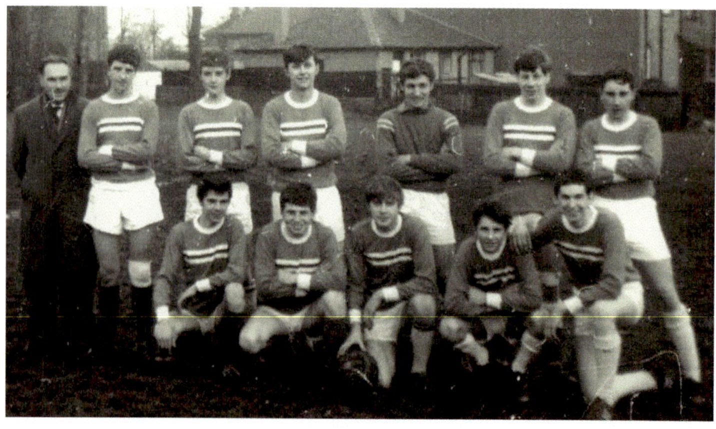

Figure 18

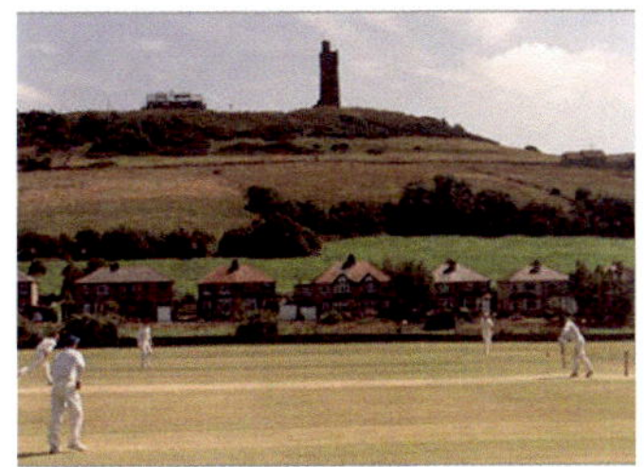

Figure 19

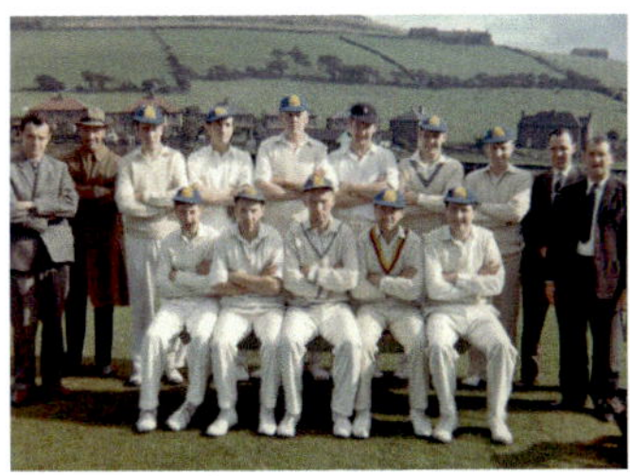

Figure 20

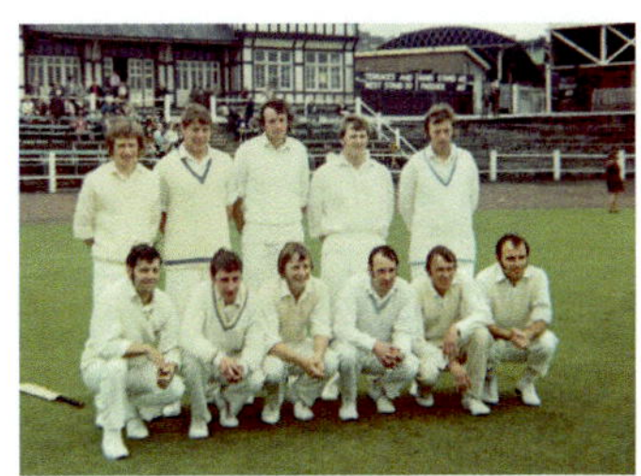

Figure 21

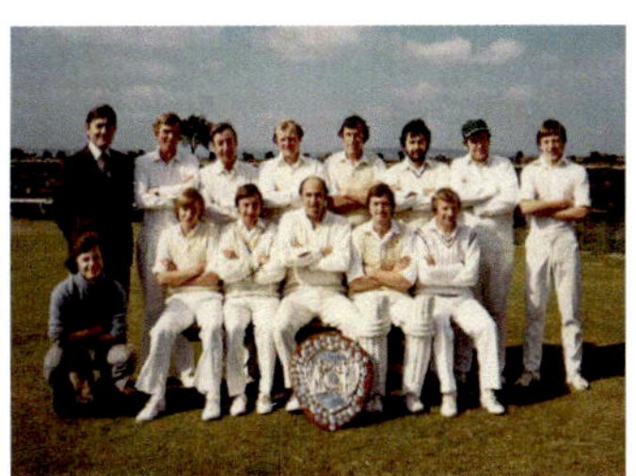

Figure 22

14·8·77

Big three make sure of Hall Bower victory

THREE tremendous performances from Ian Graham, Kevin Beaumont and Malcolm Mear won the Paddock Shield for Hall Bower.

They beat the favourites, Thongsbridge, by three wickets with two overs to spare in an exciting final of the Huddersfield League's second-eleven cup competition.

Graham snapped up three remarkable catches in helping Hall Bower restrict the home side to 156 all out, and it was enough to earn him, in the eyes of League president Alec Lodge, the Stanley Laycock Memorial Trophy for the man-of-the-match award.

Beaumont and Mear then produced two vastly different batting performances, to steer Hall Bower to victory.

Beaumont, who last year got a "duck" in the final playing for the winners, Slaithwaite, blasted 50 runs, including ten fours, in just thirteen overs out of a total of 62—4.

When he was out during a full toss straight back to left-arm quick bowler Michael Kenworthy, having made 56, all seemed lost for Hall Bower.

But Mear kept a cool head and slowly but surely inched his way toward the winning target. He was well supported by Stephen Cook, who was unbeaten on 16, when Mear made the winning runs off Kenworthy, hitting the ball on to the leg side for three.

Earlier, veteran Tommy Lynes had bowled a marathon 22.5 overs to capture five wickets for 82. He also took what was probably the most vital wicket of the day when he bowled David Walls round his legs for 17.

Walls has been in tremendous form with the bat for the first team recently, scoring almost 400 runs in six innings.

Graham's first catch came in the eighteenth over when he dived forward at mid-on to dismiss opener Michael Thornton for 23 and his second was when he plucked a full-blooded square-cut from Barry Marshall an inch from the ground.

It was his third, however, that really counted. Geoff Howard drove Lynes fiercely to mid-on and Graham raced in from the boundary and dived full length to pull off a remarkable catch.

Howard had played an extremely solid innings of 42, which included five fours and one six, and had looked capable of leading his side to a big score.

The Thongsbridge lower order batsmen could find no answer to Trevor Kaye, who replaced the economical Mear in the thirty-fourth over, and finished with four for 14 in six overs.

Figure 23

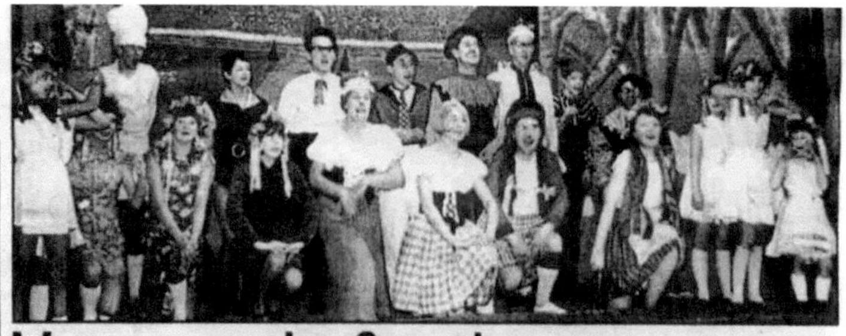

Merry souls for the moment

HE'S behind you. Berry Brow Methodist Church Pantomime Society folded in 1969 after 18 productions.

Two years previously they performed Old King Cole on the little Birch Road stage, and although our correspondent does not remember the names of the little dancers, pictured in the finale are (back row, from left): David Lockwood, Glenys Preston, Ian Whitehouse, Ian Graham, Roy Donkersley, George Boothroyd, David Bedford, Charlie Newsome

(Front kneeling): Susan Lawton, Christine Preston, Christine Lawton, Jean Donkersley, Cynthia Rouse, Susan Sykes. George Berry

Figure 24

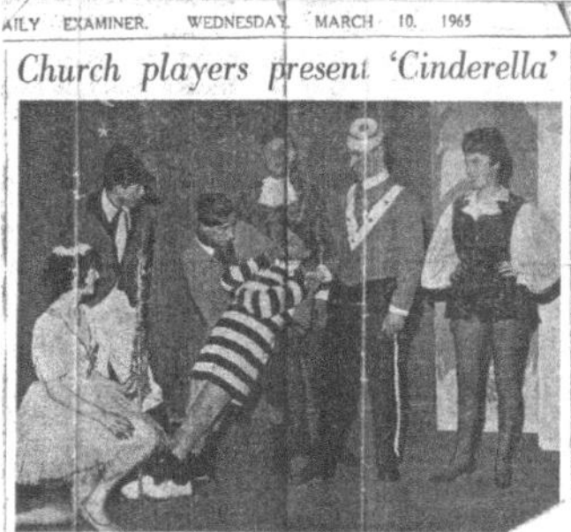

AILY EXAMINER. WEDNESDAY, MARCH 10, 1965

Church players present 'Cinderella'

THE famous story of "Cinderella" is given royal treatment by members of Berry Brow Methodist Church in the current production, which opened last night.

The show reflects gaiety and youthful enthusiasm. There is a host of tuneful songs and well-practised dance routines.

Non-stop humour is provided by Austin O'Mahony and George Berry as Buttercup and Marigold, Cinderalla's step-sisters, and Charlie Newsome and Ian Graham, as Smash and Grabbe, the broker's men.

This quartet is admirably supported by George Boothroyd, as Baron Harduppe, who also excels in his vocal numbers, and Roy Donkersley (Buttons), who gets the audience in the right mood early on with some fine patter.

The title role is played by Catherine Boothroyd, and Dandini, Prince Charming's valet, is well portrayed by Pauline Wilkinson, who combines her acting ability with a sweet singing voice.

The cast is completed by Patricia Ingham (Baroness Harduppe), David Quarmby (Prince Charming), Glenys Preston, David Lockwood, Richard Bone, Richard Poyner and David Bedford.

The chorus, which provides much more than a background to the show, comprises Christine Lawton, Jane Kaye, Susan Lawton, Christine Preston, Susan Sykes, Julia Roebuck and Janet Moore.

The show is produced by Constance M. Holmes, who also arranged the music, and additional choreography is by Marcia Heap.

The pianist is Roy Sykes and the drummer Lloyd Chappell. The show will be repeated tonight, tomorrow and on Saturday.

Pictured are (from left) Glenys Preston, David Lockwood, Ian Graham, Charlie Newsome, David Quarmby, Roy Donkersley and Pauline Wilkinson.

Figure 25

The Hepworth Iron Company Ltd.,
Head Office,
Hazlehead, Stocksbridge, Sheffield S30 5HG.
Tel: Barnsley (0226) 763561.
Telex: 54294. Fax Tel: (0226) 764827.

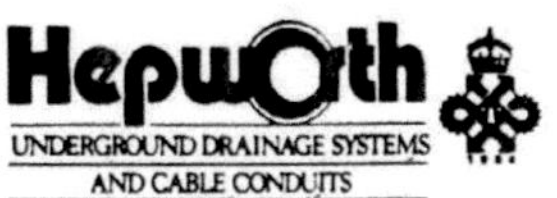

ANNOUNCEMENT

A very important part of our new Sales Organisation is to strengthen the Sales Administration function, both as a selling and service aid to the customer and an administrative and service aid to the sales force.

You are probably aware that Mr R V Hirst, our Sales Administration Manager, will be retiring at the end of this year. In order to plan for the above, I am pleased to announce that:

1. Mr Brian McCrea is promoted to Sales Administration Manager (Designate)

2. Mr Chris Hickling will be moving from Woodville to Hazlehead to take over from Brian McCrea as HQ Sales Administration Section Head

3. Mr Ian Graham, a new employee, has been appointed as Sales Office Manager of our new Northern Sales Office at Leeds.

With the exception of Mr Ian Graham, who will start his employment on Monday, 26 January, the other changes become effective from Monday, 2 February 1987.

R F Bradley
Marketing Director

21 January 1987

Registered Office: Hazlehead, Stocksbridge, Sheffield S30 5HG. Registered No. 180603 England.
A member of Hepworth Ceramic Holdings PLC.

The 1984 Queen's Award for Technological Achievement was made to the Research and Development Department of The Hepworth Iron Company Ltd. for roller kiln development.

Figure 26

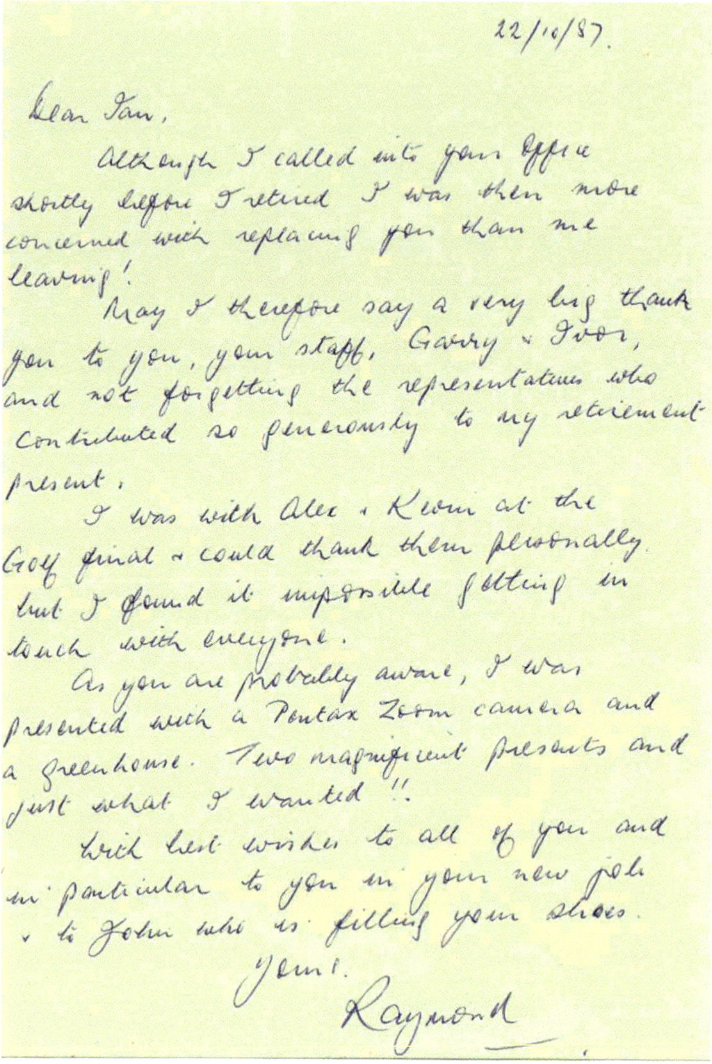

22/10/87.

Dear Ian,

Although I called into your office shortly before I retired I was then more concerned with replacing you than me leaving!

May I therefore say a very big thank you to you, your staff, Garry & Ivor, and not forgetting the representatives who contributed so generously to my retirement present.

I was with Alec & Kevin at the Golf final & could thank them personally but I found it impossible getting in touch with everyone.

As you are probably aware, I was presented with a Pentax Zoom camera and a greenhouse. Two magnificent presents and just what I wanted!!

With best wishes to all of you and in particular to you in your new job & to John who is filling your shoes.

Yours.

Raymond

Figure 27

17th December 2014

Dear Mrs Hirst

Thank you very much for seeing me last Sunday and welcoming me as you did, it was very kind and thoughtful. I understand that I may have caused a little doubt in your mind later that day. I apologise for that – it certainly was not intended, but quite understandable. Please accept my apologies for arriving without prior notice.

As I said on Sunday, I had absolutely no idea that Raymond had passed away some 15 years ago. I was, as you will recall, quite upset at the news and could not think of anything but that for the remainder of the day.

I hope you don't mind me saying so again, but Raymond was without doubt the best manager that I have ever worked for. He was also one of the nicest men one could wish to meet. I feel extremely privileged to have known him as a person, a manager and more importantly as a friend.

When I arrived home on Monday, I immediately looked at various items that I have saved and treasured over the years. One such item was a letter that Raymond sent to me immediately prior to his retirement. I have enclosed a copy of the letter for you. It is a perfect reminder of the type of gentleman that your husband was. Both you and your children must be extremely proud of him.

I will always remember Raymond and both he and the original letter will continue to be an important part of my past.

I also regret to hear from you that your son-in-law Chris passed away some time ago also. I did not know Chris very well, but I do remember him as a Representative during my second period of employment with Hepworth in the late 1980's. Please pass on my condolences to your daughter and his family. As I recall, his father Donald also worked at Hepworth during my first spell there from 1968-1974. I knew Donald quite well and had daily dealings with him.

Thank you once again for your time and the most welcome chat we had.

I sincerely hope that you all have a Merry Christmas and A Happy New Year.

Ian

Figure 28

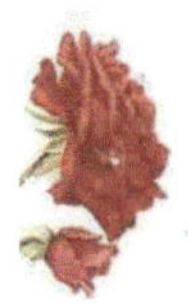

Dear Ian,

Thank you for your letter and enclosed details about Raymond. It was lovely seeing you and sharing our memories. I agree with you he was a wonderful man and I was so pleased to read your compliments.
Ray was so brave – he fought cancer but sadly lost the battle – he was so loved by the family and friends.

I do so hope your life gets settled and happy – you yourself are a kind & thoughtful gentleman.

Ruth.

Figure 29

14 THE CITIZEN, WEDNESDAY, JANUARY 12. 1994

Managing success despite recession

A MANUFACTURING firm in Gloucester has recruited a new sales and marketing manager in a bid to keep up its growing popularity.

New recruit, Andrew Halstead-Smith, started in his new post at Samson Lintels Limited, on January 1.

Mr Halstead-Smith, who has previously worked as a manager, said he wanted to build on the firm's current success.

He said: "Samson's lifeblood is the medium and small independent builders merchant.

"They want to stock quality kitemarked products at no-nonsense prices.

"Our up front discount policy has proved extremely popular.

"It is one of the reasons why our stockist network has more than doubled in size over the past couple of years."

He added: "I am confident we can double again over the next two years as we emerge from the recession."

Mr Halstead-Smith said the main priorities for Samson in the future would be customer care and delivery dates.

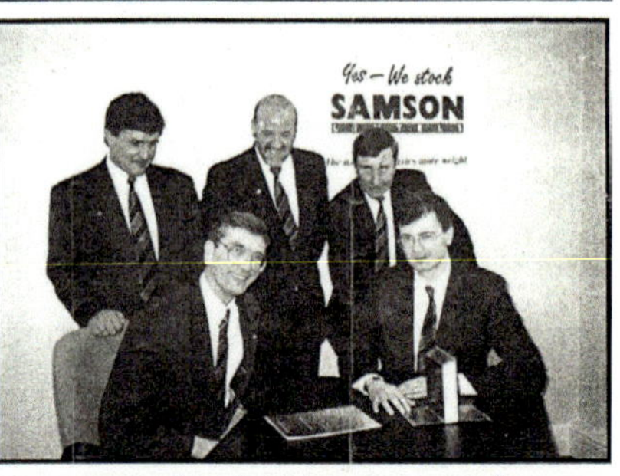

■ A new man...Andrew Halstead-Smith, the new Sales and Marketing manager at Samson Lintels, seated right with the sales team from left Steve Williams, Roger Brown, Ian Graham and Dennis Rigby, seated left.

Figure 30

I.C. Graham Esq.,
63 Towngate,
Newsome,
Huddersfield.

In Account with Eaton Smith & Downey

V.A.T. REGD. No. 183 5326 57

Solicitors

Huddersfield

17th April 1978 MMT/JH

Dr. *Cr.*

Purchase of Plot 127 Bankfield Park Ave., Taylor Hill.

Dr.	£	p
Jack Brook (Builders) Ltd. - purchase money	13,150	00
" " " " - extras as per copy account and letter herewith	232	28
NHBC - inflation "Top-up" cover premium	20	00
Kirklees MBC - legal costs anent Lease as per copy account herewith	35	00
Eaton Smith & Downey - legal costs anddisbursements anent Purchase, Mortgage and registration as per account herewith	169	25
H M Land Registry - registration fee	24	00
Stamp Duty on Lease and Counterpart	4	10
	£ 13,634	63

Cr.	£	p
Deposit paid to Jack Brook (Builders) Ltd.	150	00
Deposit paid to Eaton Smith & Downey	1,150	00
Halifax Building Society - Mortgage advance	12,000	00
Balance due from you	334	63
	£ 13,634	63

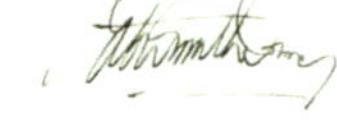

Figure 31

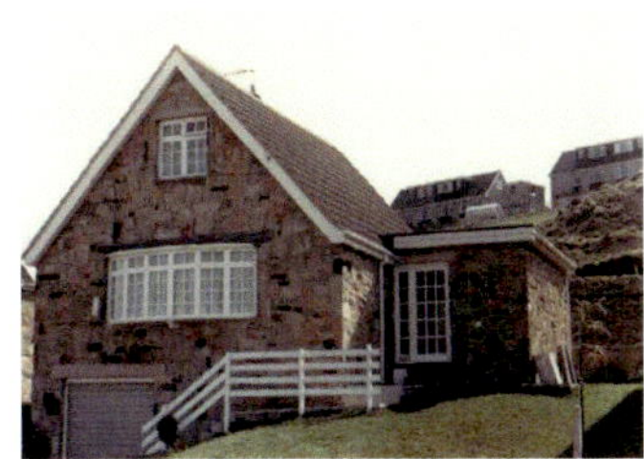

Figure 32

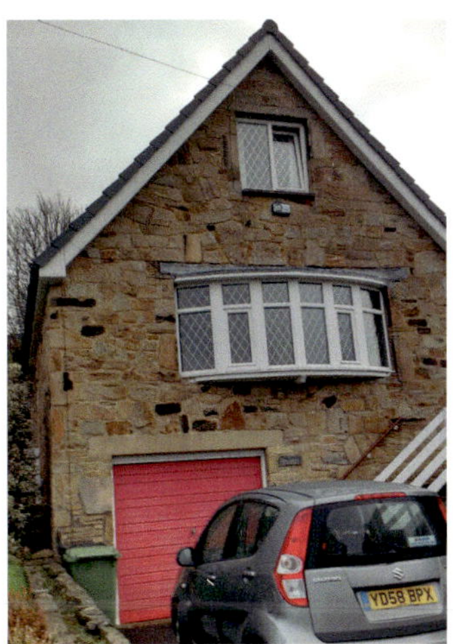

Figure 33

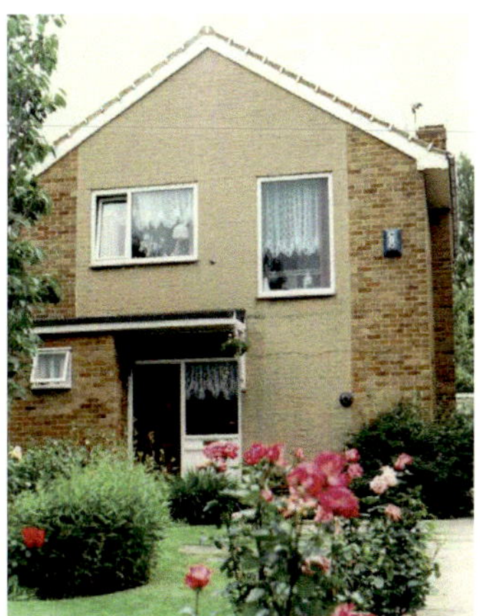

Figure 34

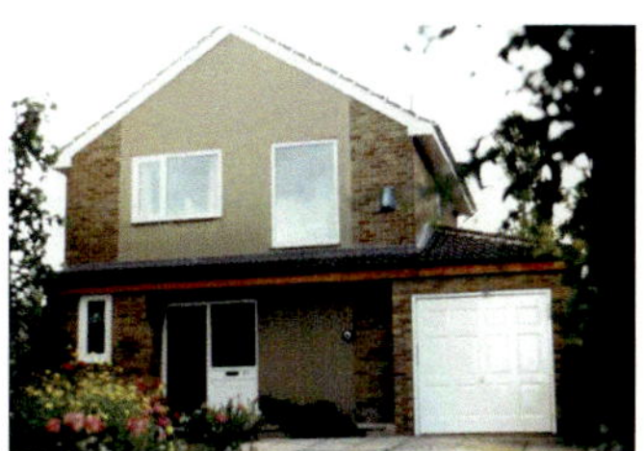

Figure 35

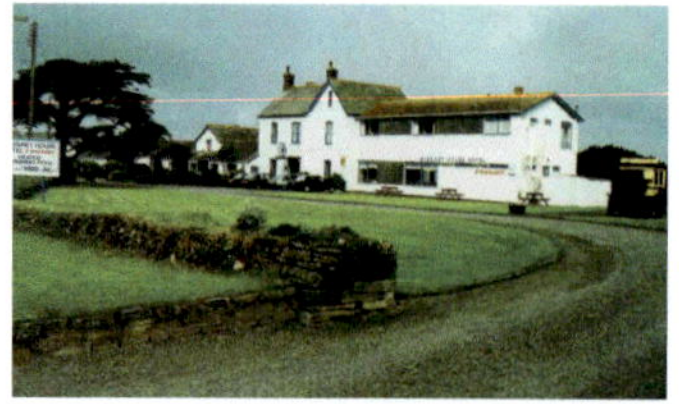

Figure 36

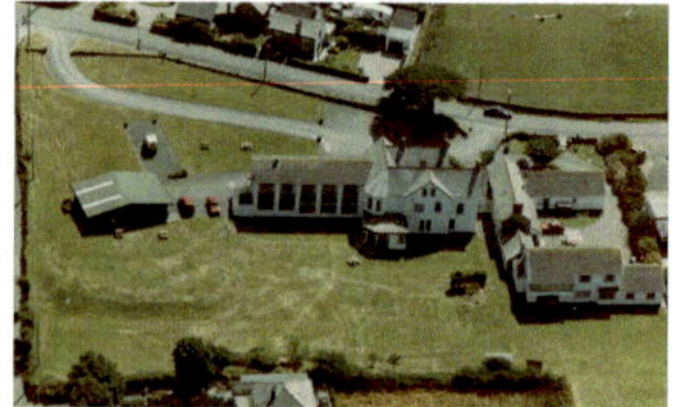

Figure 37

Bossiney House Hotel
Tintagel, Cornwall, PL34 0AX
Telephone 01840 770240 Fax 01840 770501

Sir Francis Drake
M.P. 1583

Tintagel Castle

13th May 1996

Speake Medley Ltd
Egerton House
Town Street
Rawdon
Leeds
LS19 6QA

F.A.O. Mr D Speake

Dear Derrick

Re: Cannings & Graham Household Insurances

Thank you for your letters of today concerning the above.

Please go ahead with the policy for Cannings as per your letter and the Fire Mark Policy with Sun Alliance for ourselves. I am inclined to suggest ignoring the Travel Insurance but hoping that we will be able to go abroad in the winter I think that it would be better to take it up at the extra price of £90. Therefore please go ahead as paragraph 2 of your letter.

Please include both within your standing order details as discussed.

Thank you for your advice yet again.

Yours sincerely

Ian.

Ian C Graham

AA RAC ★★

APPROVED

Figure 38

BOSSINEY HOUSE HOTEL
Here
cooks
and serves
the Boss
himself personal
Tintagel NORTH Cornwall
During the week 5.-12.6.1999 he always
had an open ear for our wishes.
A Lot of thanks to you and your
family

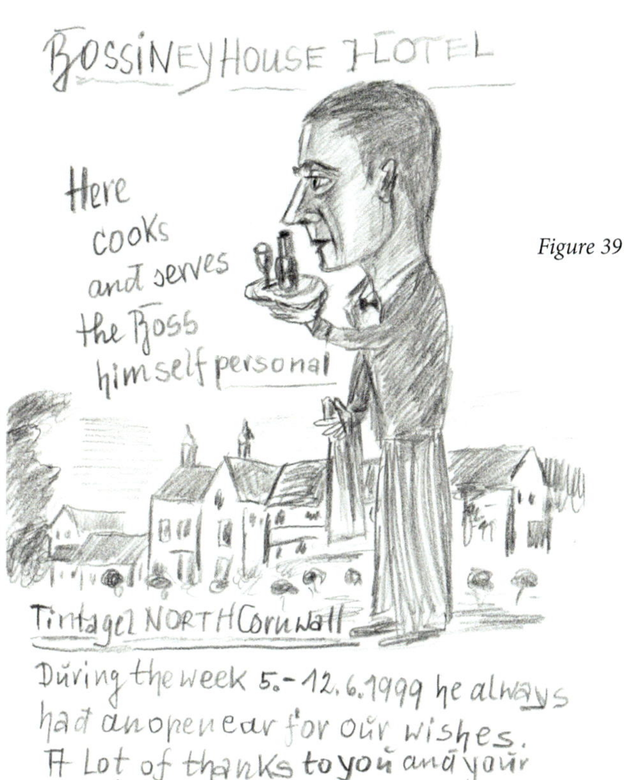

Figure 39

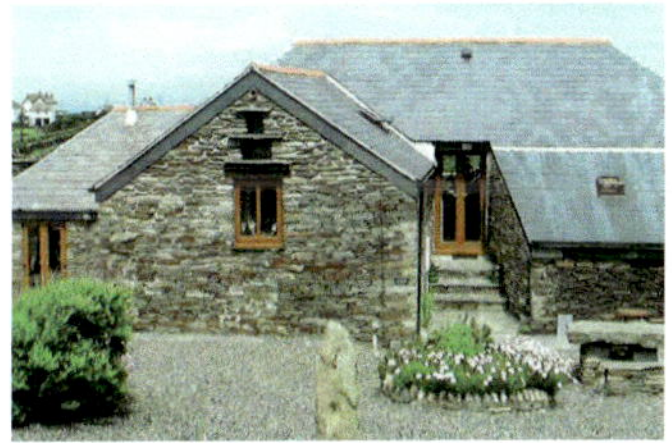

Figure 40

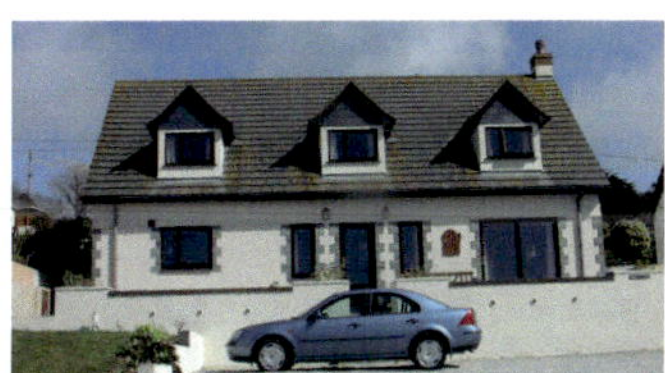

Figure 41

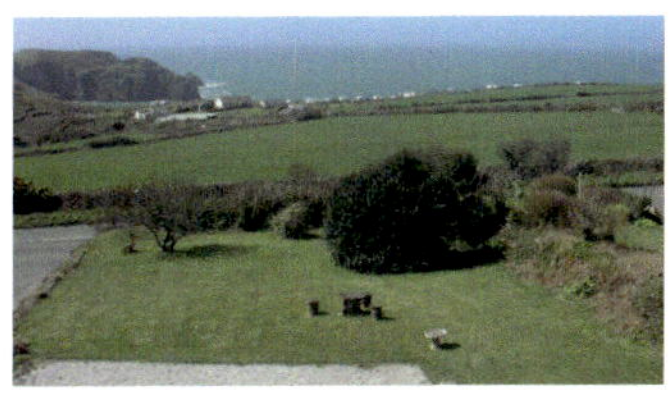

Figure 42

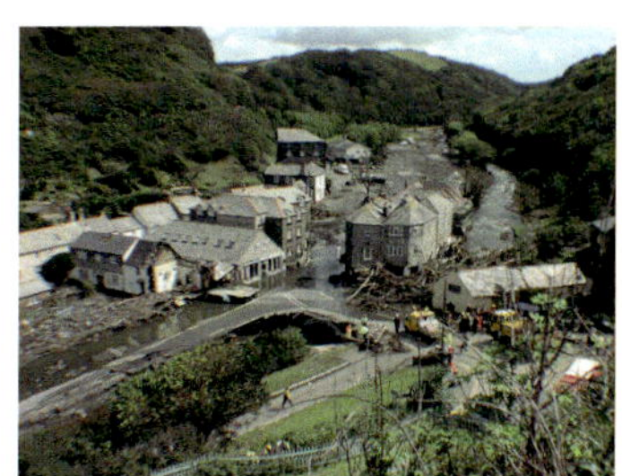

Figure 43

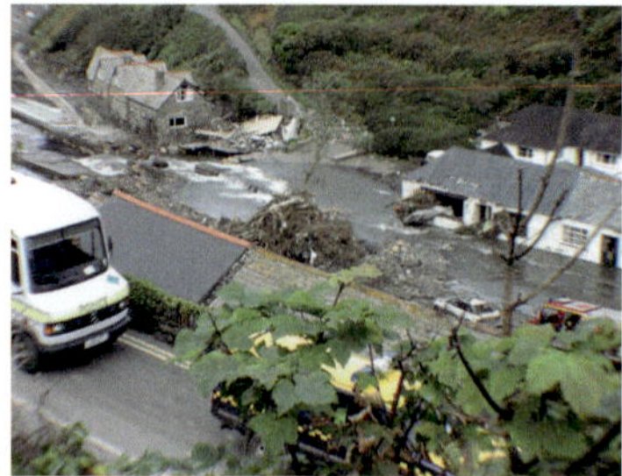

Figure 44

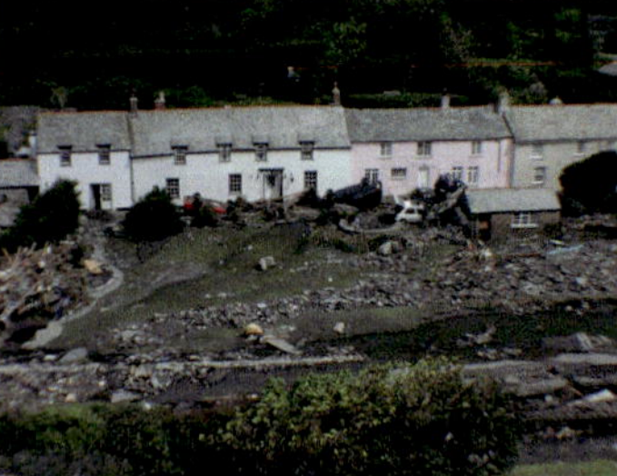

Figure 45

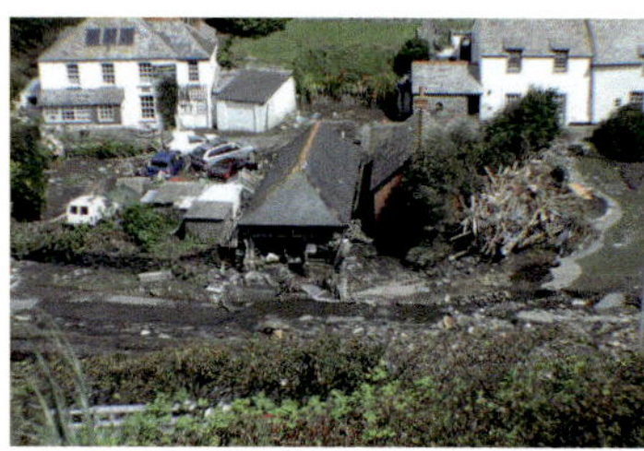

Figure 46

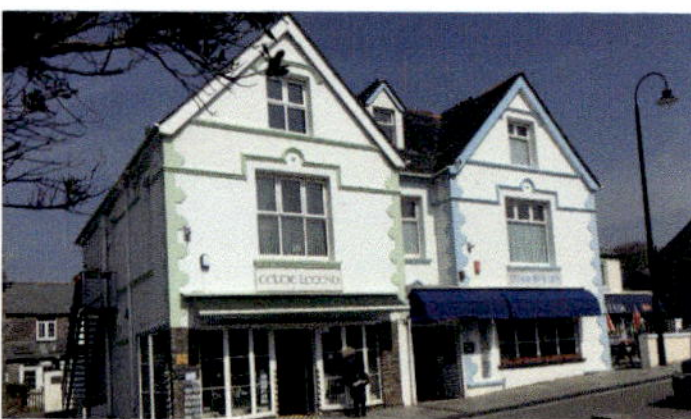

Figure 47

Dear Mr Craham,

Thank you for your letter dated the 23rd July 2015. We are pleased to hear that you have made a full recovery and we are sorry for any distress that you may have suffered during this unfortunate incidence.

As requested, we have discussed this at our monthly clinical team meeting, which is attended by all Drs and nurses at the practice. We have taken on board the lessons that you have presented so eloquently in your letter. As I am sure you are aware when a Doctor makes a diagnosis there is always a balance of risks to take into account and sometimes without all the specialist tests and equipment available it is difficult to make an accurate diagnosis; both a stroke and a retinal detachment can present in very similar ways.

Obviously we have all taken on board the lessons to be learned and wish you all the best in the future.

Yours sincerely

Drs Garrod & Abbott

Figure 49

Dear Graham

<u>Re: My appointment of 9th July 2015</u>

On the above date I visited Tintagel Surgery requesting an emergency consultation with a doctor as I was experiencing an unusual eye problem. Due to the surgery being busy I was requested to attend the surgery waiting room at 11am to wait to be attended to.

I was duly seen by Dr , who after examining and questioning me as to the symptoms experienced by me a few days before, came to the conclusion that I may have had a small stroke. The symptoms I experienced were in my left eye and the weekend before had been seeing dark "bubbles" in my sight. On the Tuesday I lost approximately 25% of my sight in the bottom right hand side of my eye. On the Wednesday this had increased to approximately 50%. In the top half of my eye sight I could see light only and could not focus on anything at all with this eye.

Dr informed me that she would contact the hospital stroke unit requesting they make an appointment to examine me. In the meantime she informed me that I would not be able to drive my car as it was necessary for her to inform me that I would not be insured as instructed by DVLA. Consequently I have not driven since.

The following day, Friday, the stroke unit attempted to contact me at home by telephone to arrange an appointment. They were unable to do so as I was at work in the shop. They eventually contacted me at the shop at approximately 4.40pm and offered me an appointment either at Bodmin on Tuesday 14th July or at Treliske the following day Saturday 11th July. I originally requested the Bodmin appointment but a few minutes later changed it to the Treliske appointment for the following day.

My youngest daughter Nicola, along with her partner and son, drove me to Truro for the 1pm appointment. I was given an ECG and had an Ultrasound examination of the veins in my neck and asked to await the arrival of the consultant on duty for further consultation. When seen I was immediately informed that it was not a stroke that I had suffered but an obvious optical problem. She also informed me that my GP should have arranged for me to see the Emergency Eye Clinic immediately and not the stroke unit. She then made arrangements for me to be seen by an ophthalmic consultant that afternoon in the Emergency Eye Clinic, a Mr George.

The clinic was very busy with patients and I was attended to after an approximate 2 hour wait. I was again given an ECG, had a sight test and had various drops put in to both eyes. When Mr George then examined me he informed me that I had a badly detached retina and required almost immediate surgery. He contacted an eye specialist, Mr Murjaneh, and an appointment to operate was made for 9am Sunday 12th July. Mr George also stated that my GP should have diagnosed that the problem was with the eye and not a stroke.

Prior to the operation, Mr Murjaneh gave my eyes a thorough examination and informed me that due to the few days delay in the diagnosis, the operation may not be totally successful. He was also of the opinion that my GP had made the wrong initial decision.

I was duly operated on and allowed home later that afternoon and requested to return the following lunchtime for further check ups. Mr Murjaneh informed me that the operation appeared to be a success but would see me again on Monday 20th July for a further check up. Following this check up, I was much relieved to be informed that the operation was indeed successful and that the retina was now back in place and that I should gradually gain full sight over the next few weeks. An appointment is being made for my next check up in approximately 4 weeks time. In the meantime I have been advised that if anything does not seem right with my eye, I should contact the Emergency Eye Clinic immediately.

The reason for me advising you of the above is that I would hate for someone else to go through the same situation. I feel that my unfortunate experience should perhaps be made known to the group practice in order that it does not occur again.

Eye sight is probably the most precious "gift" of all and to lose it must be devastating.

Kind regards

Ian

Figure 48

20 March 2017

Dear Mr Graham

The Partners have discussed your appeal to stay registered with Bottreaux Surgery.

Their imperative is to provide appropriate and safe health care to all the patients registered with the Practice. In this instance, there is unanimous agreement that your new address is too far outside of the core practice area to be able to achieve this. You will therefore need to register with another Practice.

Your nearest GP Practices are:

Dr Andrew Garrod, The Medical Centre, Church Field, Camelford, Cornwall PL32 9YT

Dr Tony Nash, The Medical Centre, Church Field, Camelford, Cornwall PL32 9YT

I appreciate that this is not the response that you were hoping for, but the Partners have carefully considered all the information you provided.

Yours sincerely

Business Manager

Figure 50

History

Presenting complaint or issue:
Referred for procedure: 12/03/19
History: Dgn: Left hip OA.
Plan: Left hip replacement.

Mr Graham was referred for the left hip pain. It affects his everyday activities and also disturbs him occasionally at night. He localises pain in the groin and in the buttock and it can be referred down to the thigh. He does not feel any pain in the right hip. He underwent stroke in the past and there is right sided weakness mostly affecting his upper limb.

Clinical summary

Planned procedure:
PRIMARY HYBRID PROSTHETIC REPLACEMENT OF HIP JOINT USING CEMENTED FEMORAL COMPONENT

Laterality:
Left

Clinical examination:
X-rays confirm osteoarthrosis in left hip joint with loss of joint space, subchondral sclerosis, cysts and marginal osteophytes.
No fixed flexion but significantly restricted flexion, abduction and rotational movements.

Case type:
Inpatient

Anaesthetic:
Spinal + Sedation

Follow Up Note: 9 JUL 2019
Patient was seen today following a left total hip replacement on 10/05/2019. He is happy with the outcome of his surgery and mobilises well unaided. He manages residual pain well, his surgical scar healed well and he has a good ROM. I reviewed his post-operative x-ray and found no abnormalities. I encouraged him to continue with exercises to further strengthen the hip. The pain he had in his right hip has settled down totally and we have agreed that treatment to the right hip seems unnecessary at this point in time. He is discharged today and will be followed up in one year.

Plan and requested actions

Actions for healthcare professional: 12/03/19
Mr Graham was offered hip replacement. All risks and possible complications such as: infection, deep vein thrombosis, pulmonary embolism, fracture, dislocation, nerve/vessel injury, leg length discrepancy and early loosening of implants were explained to the patient and listed in the informed consent form which patient signed. Booked accordingly.

Figure 51

discussion between the two of them. That Steve was a married man with young children and there would be no way in which his father would react except to offer himself for redundancy. I then told Michael that in my opinion this should be his decision to make and any other way should not even be considered. It should be his responsibility alone.

The next day I was informed that Ben and Steve had been informed of Michael's decision. I was right – Ben offered himself as the sacrificial lamb – there was never any doubt in my mind that the outcome would be any different. I still maintain to this day that Michael should have made the decision himself and not left it to them to decide their future between themselves.

Not long afterwards, Catnic made another, much larger decision in respect of Samson, but this time in respect of our manufacturing facility based within the John Carr premises in Gloucester. The manufacturing unit was to be transferred in its entirety to another company within the Catnic group, Frederick Jones Ltd, who also manufactured steel lintels and was based in Oswestry, Shropshire, close to the North Wales border. Frederick Jones manufactured really heavy-duty lintels and was considered to be the best manufacturer in the country in respect of the heavy-duty lintel. It didn't take long to move the machinery and stock to Oswestry, but the Samson sales office remained in Gloucester.

A lot had happened during the three years or so that I had been with Samson in addition to the above mentioned. We had developed sales to an extent that we employed an internal sales clerk, Mike Flynn, and a sales representative was appointed to cover the south-east, Roger Brown, I continued to cover the north of England and North Wales and occasionally Scotland, Dennis the midlands, and Steve, South Wales and south-west England. Michael was available to make visits out of areas uncovered and to assist the four of us as and when required. Jon of course was very busy looking after everything to do within the office. Phil moved to the Catnic factory in Caerphilly following the manufacturing transfer to Oswestry.

In November 1993, Catnic had quite a large stand at the NEC for the usual building exhibition and Samson were invited to take a section of it. Michael and Jon planned our part in it, and Dennis, Steve, Roger and me were appointed to represent Samson on the stand for the duration of the exhibition. Just before the exhibition and totally unbeknown to us, Michael had been offered the position of Managing Director of Selflock Ltd, a supplier of ductile, cast iron and steel manhole covers and frames. As mentioned earlier, Michael had worked for Selflock in the 1980s when they were situated in South Wales. Selflock were now owned by a French company called Norinco and now situated in Misterton, a village just outside Doncaster, South Yorkshire. He had decided to accept the position and tendered his notice to Peter Morgan, which was reluctantly accepted. When Michael told me of his decision, he suggested that I apply for the now vacant position and that I would be a perfect replacement for him. I duly did and, both during the exhibition and over dinners at the hotel we were staying at, was casually interviewed by David Hey, who had recently been appointed Sales and Marketing Director of Catnic in place of Geoff Hirons.

Apparently, there were two of us being considered for the position, Andrew Halstead-Smith, who was employed in the marketing department at the Catnic head office in Caerphilly, and me. David informed us both that a decision would be made regarding Michael's replacement within the week following the exhibition. I was looking forward in anticipation to being appointed and had been informed by Michael that I was considered favourite for the job. It came as a big disappointment when David Hey rang me a few days later to say that he had decided to appoint Andrew to the position. He also informed me that I was considered a valuable asset, by both himself and Peter Morgan, to the Samson future and that he would appreciate my continued work on their behalf even though he knew I would be feeling very disappointed at the decision.

Michael continued as sales manager at Samson for the next few weeks, finally leaving us at the closure for the Christmas break. We resumed work following Christmas and New Year and Andrew commenced his employment as sales manager based at the offices in Gloucester. The first sales meeting he held was in the second week of the New Year. We had, of course, spoken by telephone a number of times, and I, as had the other representatives, assured him that we would continue under his leadership as we had done in the past for Michael. During that first meeting it had been arranged for a trade publication to write a short column regarding the new appointment, for the five of us to be photographed together with the article appearing in the publication on 12th January 1994. We all duly continued working hard in our respective areas, and sales increased over the next few months, as we had forecast.

During the summer of 1994 I had been visiting customers in the north Lincolnshire area when I received an unexpected telephone call from Michael Miles whilst travelling back home. After the usual pleasantries he asked if I could perhaps give him some advice concerning a problem he had. Naturally I said that I would do my best and he asked me to meet him at a hotel in Garforth just off the M62 between Leeds and Wakefield. I arrived at 4pm to find Michael waiting in the car park in his car. We went inside, ordered drinks and sat down to hear what advice I might be able to offer him. He went on to tell me that his commercial director had been diagnosed with a terminal illness and had unfortunately been forced to relinquish his post with immediate effect. Michael then asked me if I might be able to recommend a suitable replacement to fill the position, living within a reasonable distance of Misterton. I jokingly replied that I was the only person I knew. His reply was that that was the answer he was hoping to hear. He went on to explain the requirements of the position, that I would be appointed as commercial manager on a salary of £25,000 p.a. with a company car and the usual expenses. However, the appointment would be subject to meeting Richard Keighley, the financial director of Selflock.

I was very pleased and somewhat excited that Michael had approached me, and we arranged a meeting with Richard for the following week. The meeting with Richard was almost like a full-blown interview, and I wasn't really prepared for that. After the interview Michael told me that he would ring me the following day with more information, along with Richard's comments. The next day I was offered the position of commercial manager by Michael but at the lower salary of £23,000 p.a., which was apparently instigated by Richard. I was informed that the salary would be reviewed after a trial period of twelve months. After thinking about it for a few moments I agreed to accept it.

The next day I informed Andrew Halstead-Smith of the offer and that I would be tendering my notice to him in writing. A short while later he rang me back to inform me that they were very reluctant to accept it but were not in a position to compete with the offer from Selflock. During the next month I continued to give my all to Samson. I had very much enjoyed the four years with the company and, I must admit, was quite sad to be leaving. When the time came to hand over the company car and the records, etc., that I had compiled during my time with Samson, I was invited to the office in Gloucester for a couple of days. Andrew arranged a final meal with my former colleagues and I was presented with a commemorative glass tankard as a thank you for my efforts over the time I had been with them. Samson arranged and paid for my journey home by rail.

Just prior to commencing employment with Selflock, Michael rang me asking if I would do him a favour. My predecessor's company car, a BMW 5 Series Saloon, was a leased vehicle and still had a few months to go prior to the end of the term. He asked me if I would mind taking that vehicle on for the remainder of the lease, after which a new Ford Mondeo Saloon would be made available to me. Even though my taxable benefit in kind would be greater for the BMW than the Mondeo, I agreed to take it on, as it would save Selflock having to pay for the remainder of the lease in addition to the cost of a new Mondeo. It turned out to be the best car I had ever driven up to then, and I had driven quite a few different models over the years, most of them company cars. After I had been driving it for about four months it developed a problem with the automatic gearbox. The problem was diagnosed to be quite expensive to repair and it was suggested I carry on with the problem, which thankfully wasn't dangerous. Had it been I would of course have rejected the request.

Selflock was originally founded in the 1950s and was based in Cwmbran, South Wales, manufacturing cast iron manhole covers and frames, gully gratings and frames, and ancillary products. They were responsible for designing and manufacturing the self-locking and self-levelling range of products, hence the company name of Selflock. In 1986, they were acquired by the French company Norinco Group, initially continuing to operate in Cwmbran but later moving to the Misterton site near Doncaster, South Yorkshire. In 2000 Selflock were renamed Norinco UK. In 2004 an American company, East Jordan Iron Works, based in Michigan, acquired the whole of the Norinco Group, and this company became known simply as E J in 2012. The various subsidiary companies, Selflock, Norinco, etc. are now known as E J UK, etc.

It took time to settle in to life at Selflock, which I found to be totally different to anything I had done before. Unfortunately,

Michael didn't help the situation, as he had, in my opinion, changed the way he managed people. When at Samson he had allowed people, within reason, to make their own way in how they developed their positions and gave them the freedom to make decisions. He was obviously at hand to help and rectify things if needed. But at Selflock I found that virtually everything had to pass "over his desk". Quotations to customers, orders received, purchasing of stock – just about everything had to be approved by him.

In addition to Michael and Richard, the other members of staff were Anthony Dance, Andrew Collins and Andy Rowland, all based at the Misterton offices, along with the representatives of the company, David Oakley, Arthur Goosen, Mike Thornton and Stuart Young, all of whom worked from home in their respective areas of operation.

All of the manhole covers and gully gratings, etc., that were stocked at our premises in Misterton were manufactured in ductile or cast iron at our parent company's headquarters and factory near Paris in France. We had to order products from them every month, which were shipped in by road transport. Whether we were overstocked with any items or not, we HAD to place monthly orders of twenty tonnes. I found this to be somewhat ridiculous, but it was written in stone! If we were overstocked on items (and we quite often were), we had to sell products even at a slight loss in order to make room for more. Selflock also manufactured a range of steel access covers at our Misterton premises specially made to order. Andy Rowland, who also designed units for specific requirements to the customer's request, managed the steel department. He and I had a confrontation just after I took delivery of the new Mondeo. He also ran a company vehicle, a Citroen Saloon, which to be fair was not in the same class as the Mondeo. He was extremely vehement towards me because of the car I had been allotted, which, as I say, was much nicer than his. I informed him as calmly as I could that I had been given a short list of vehicles to choose from, which included the Citroen model that he had, but I had chosen the Mondeo after careful consideration. I also told him that if he wasn't happy about it to see Michael and not take it out on me. After this we seemed to get on quite well, believe it or not.

The other members of the sales office consisted of Anthony Dance, who was primarily our customers' main point of contact if requiring steel access covers and frames, and Andrew Collins, who dealt with all ductile and cast iron products that we supplied. Both were responsible for the initial dealing with enquiries for the products and administration and implementation of orders received. A secretary was also employed.

Part of my remit was to spend time out on the road with our representatives, seeing customers throughout their regions and helping them to achieve their objectives. This I hardly ever did, as I felt that I was being kept in the office "learning" the Selflock ways. Primarily the supermarket chains – Sainsbury's, Asda, Tesco, Morrisons, Waitrose and Safeway – used a product line that Selflock were trying hard to break in to. The product being an access cover manufactured in steel with a brass edge and used throughout the supermarket stores to gain access to the service ducts that carried the cables, etc. from the checkout areas to the offices. Howe Green Ltd currently manufactured the covers used by them all to a very high standard, with excellent tolerances and an extremely aesthetic finish. The steel department at Selflock was unable to manufacture the product due to the requirement of the brass edge, and due to this, a company in the midlands was appointed to manufacture the Selflock equivalent which was named Alumatic on their behalf. The finished product, however, was nowhere near as good as the Howe Green cover. This did not deter Michael Miles, who was determined that the product should be a success.

Our Scotland representative, Stuart Young, was appointed the main salesman responsible for the success (or failure) in the UK sales of the alumatic cover. As hard as he tried (and he did try very hard), the cover was a virtual complete failure. In my opinion, not only was it lacking in quality but, the pricing was also high compared to the Howe Green product in comparison.

During 1995, a new airport was being built in Hong Kong, and Michael spent a couple of weeks over there trying to achieve orders for a heavy-duty range of multiple covers and frames that Norinco manufactured at the factory near Paris. They were to be used on and around the runways at the airport, and it was absolutely essential that they were of top quality, capable of carrying a great weight and able to stand the pressures put upon them by aircraft of all types, along with varying weather conditions. The main competitor to Selflock/Norinco was a manufacturer based in Dover called Elkington Gatic, who were and still are market leaders of this type of cover and frame. Now known simply as Gatic Ltd, the company is still operating successfully from its factory based in Dover.

Whilst Michael was away in Hong Kong, he left me in charge of the sales personnel but insisted that I fax him every day with details of orders and enquiries received, along with quotations to customers prior to them being dealt with or mailed out to customers. The monthly stock order to Norinco had to be seen by him before being faxed to them. Now in my opinion, we were overstocked on almost everything and I informed Michael so. As mentioned earlier it was a condition specified by Norinco that we HAD to purchase twenty tonnes of castings every month irrespective of our current stockholding. Michael made it absolutely clear to me that an order would be placed accordingly. During the time he was away I chaired the monthly sales meeting with the sales force and was instructed to fax the minutes of the meeting to him in Hong Kong immediately afterwards. The decision as to who was to be the successful supplier of the airport contract would not be made by the Hong Kong authorities for some time, and although Michael had worked very hard on the project, he had no alternative but to wait for the decision to be made.

That decision was made following my leaving Selflock, and I understand that Gatic was the eventual successful supplier. I have very recently been informed (over twenty-one years later), that Michael was, however, successful in securing a substantial order for Selflock to supply a quantity of similar castings to Manchester Airport shortly afterwards.

Just before Christmas 1995 it was time for all the staff to have their annual performance review. This was a new experience for me, as I had not previously worked for a company who held this practice. Michael duly reviewed my last few months' performance, which ended with me being informed that my performance was totally unacceptable to him. He informed me that he expected me to obtain orders for the alumatic range of covers within the following few weeks or I would have my employment with Selflock terminated. I was given a letter to this effect on our last working day before the Christmas break. What a bombshell that was, particularly being on that particular day – it reminded me of a similar decision he had made whilst general manager at Samson Lintels. Needless to say, it was somewhat heartbreaking to inform my wife Heather that evening.

On return to work following the Christmas and New Year break I informed Michael that I was not at all happy with the ultimatum, particularly with the alumatic product being, in my opinion, substandard in quality in comparison to the Howe Green product that was market leader and the one most used throughout the country. Following more discussions over the next few days it was mutually agreed that I would be made redundant effective from 1st February 1996 and would receive three months' salary in lieu of notice. During that time, I would be allowed to keep a company vehicle, not the Mondeo, but was expected to pay for any petrol that I used.

That was the end of my Selflock career and a totally new one was about to commence, which will appear later in this story.

Chapter 5

Married Life and Family Beginnings

DURING 1975 YOU will recall that whilst I was working at A W Lumb & Co Ltd, I met a young lady called Heather Cannings who was shortly to become a very special part of my life. I found Heather to be very attractive and it wasn't long before I plucked up the courage to ask her out. I say plucked up the courage because I thought that due to our age difference of very close to ten years, I was not at all sure that she would be interested in someone so much older than she was. Additionally, of course, there were her parents' thoughts to be considered. I needn't have worried too much, as we seemed to hit it off and over the next couple of years or so spent almost all of our spare time together, including holidays with Heather and her parents and occasionally, her grandma and grandad, Edith and Frank Hartley, and her Aunty Anne.

One of their favourite places to spend a few days' break was a cottage in a very small village in North Wales called Tan Lan, which is situated between Portmadog and Ffestiniog. We all spent time there on a number of occasions and it was an excellent place to relax and enjoy the clean Welsh air and countryside. If I remember correctly, the stream that ran through the cottage garden from the hillside beyond, actually supplied all of the water used by the holidaymakers using the cottage. That was certainly something we weren't used to back at home in Yorkshire. The local sheep also used the stream!

One particular winter holiday we had there was one to remember. Heather's parents and their three Dalmations travelled in one car, and Heather and I in mine. The weather was somewhat atrocious whilst we were travelling there and when we arrived at the entrance of the lane leading to the cottage, we were more than surprised to find that the stream had flooded very badly, and the lane was completely submerged in floodwater. It was impossible to even consider driving our cars through the water, which was so deep that you couldn't see the contours or direction of the lane. The cottage gardens were also under water. To our very pleasant surprise, and relief, a local farmer gave us all a ride, the dogs running behind above the water line, in his tractor from the main road, along the flooded lane and right to the cottage entrance. The next morning the flood had subsided enough for us to bring our cars from the main road to the cottage, and following our dramatic start, we eventually enjoyed our few days' break.

Heather and her parents lived in a detached dormer bungalow situated in Southfield Close, Horbury, a small town situated just outside the city of Wakefield. Her grandparents lived around a mile away in an area of Horbury known as The Avenues, which was only a short car ride or walk away. A number of other relations, aunties, uncles and cousins, also lived in and around The Avenues, and they were quite a close-knit family. Unfortunately, in October 1977 Heather's grandma, Edith Hartley, passed away unexpectedly. I don't remember the circumstances or much at all about the funeral but do recall quite emphatically something that occurred during the family get-together following the funeral which was held at Heathers parents' house.

We had not been there long that I felt the need to visit the bathroom, which was situated downstairs close to the side entrance door of the house. I was washing my hands when something made me look up over my right shoulder towards the bathroom ceiling at one corner of the room. Looking down at me (a shiver is going down my neck and back as I am typing this) was Edith's face with the broadest smile you could imagine. I looked away and almost immediately looked back again to see her still smiling down at me. She disappeared a few seconds later, leaving me to think things through. I am absolutely certain to this very day that it was not something that I had imagined or could be put down to alcohol, as I hadn't had one single drink. I thought about it for a few moments before returning to the room full of family. A little later I decided to tell Heather and her parents about it, who in turn told Frank of my experience. He later told Heather's parents that he was extremely happy and pleased that it had happened and was very pleased that his late wife, Edith, had been smiling.

Now I fully realise that reading something like this probably brings a few thoughts to people's minds. He imagined it! He had been drinking! He's made it up! Well – as I point out above – I am certain to this very day that it DID happen!

Heather's granddad, Frank, passed away in May 1986 and her Aunty Anne, who never married, still lives at the same house on The Avenues in Horbury. Many of Heather's other relatives continue to live on The Avenues also.

Heather and I continued our courtship over the next couple of years or so and spent most of our spare time together. We were steadily saving up in the hope of building enough savings to put down a deposit on a mortgage if things worked out that way between us. We both continued working at Lumb's for the next year or so but after a time decided that it may be better for our relationship if Heather looked to work elsewhere. We were literally spending all day (every day) and most evenings together, which caused us to occasionally argue and fall out with each other, which neither of us wanted to happen. Consequently, Heather applied for and was successful in being offered a job at another builder's merchants, Cawoods Building Materials, situated in Wakefield.

Heather duly started work there one Monday morning, but things were not to her liking and she decided not to return there after lunch – on the first day! I recall her telling me that during the morning she was asked to make drinks for her fellow colleagues in the office. What she did not know was that there was no running water in the office and that she had to go into the stockyard to fill the kettle with water from a standpipe! Furthermore, she was expected to wash the dirty mugs out at the standpipe that had been left dirty over the weekend! That was that – end of new job – and I don't blame her at all; I would have done the same.

Shortly after that unfortunate episode Heather saw a position for a receptionist advertised at a company called Eurocopy (Great Britain) Ltd based in East Ardsley, just a short distance from Wakefield. She applied for the position, attended an interview and was offered the job all within a few days, remaining there and enjoying her new job for the next few years. Heather's mum, Pat, used to drive her to work each day, and either Pat, her dad John or I would pick her up after work in order to take her back home. We continued our courtship over the next few months and spent most evenings and weekends together.

I was still playing football and cricket in Huddersfield, and most Wednesday evenings during the football season were spent training and Saturday afternoons playing. In summer it was cricket and Tuesday evenings were practice nights and Saturday afternoons playing. The cricket matches invariably did not finish until 8.00 or even 9.00pm, but I would go to Heather's after the matches incessantly. Now, Heather was not really a sports fan at all but understood that I was, and it was not a problem for us. I don't recall Heather ever watching me playing football, but she did occasionally come to cricket matches with me. Not a lot – but she did.

The one evening exception was Friday night. Friday night had been "lads' night" for as long as I was old enough to legally go to the pub. I say "lads" loosely, as it was always with my youngest brother Glyn and our best friend Trevor Ellis, and we always stayed locally in either Berry Brow or Newsome. Our regular watering holes were The Railway, The Golden Fleece or Liberal Club in Berry Brow or The Wellington in Newsome. We very rarely went anywhere else and even more rarely did we venture out by car.

In addition to spending occasional holidays with Heather and her parents, Heather and I once spent a few days together on holiday at Lynton and Lynmouth on the north coast of Devon. This was, of course, with her parents' permission, and naturally, I had booked separate rooms! From memory I don't recall the weather being all that good, it was quite a cloudy few days, but it didn't stop us getting about a bit and enjoying our few days together.

When we were still working at Lumb's we occasionally had lunches together, and one particular lunch remains well entrenched in my memory. We had gone to The Kaye Arms, a pub restaurant at Grange Moor, a small village between Wakefield and Huddersfield, which was owned by a man called Stuart Coldwell and his wife. I had quite frequently had lunches there previously, usually with David Briggs, Malcolm Roberts and David Buddery, and even Arthur and David Lumb on occasions, so knew the establishment quite well. The meals were always good, and the pub was well kept and was a very popular venue.

There we were sat having a drink after having had our lunch, chatting away and minding our own business, when Stuart Coldwell came to our table and told us to stop "canoodling" and me to stop touching Heather's legs under the table, as we were embarrassing and upsetting other customers, one of whom had complained about our behaviour. Now, we were not doing anything of the sort, never had done, and that sort of behaviour was not in either of our lives and I told him so. I also asked him who had complained and suggested that whoever it was should approach us and repeat the complaint, which was totally unfounded. I also reminded him that I had been a regular customer over the last two or three years or so, and if he was not prepared to believe that we were behaving without reproach, we would not be returning to his premises again. He obviously chose not to accept what I had said because he turned around and walked away without another word, and we immediately left the premises. It was months before we set foot in The Kaye Arms again; in fact, it was quite a few years, but a little more of this later!

We continued our courtship over the next few months, and in late summer in 1977 we decided to get married to each other and spend the rest of our lives together. Shortly after we got engaged, we started talking about where we might live. My preference was naturally in the area that I was used to, and Heather's preference was her natural area – surprise, surprise!

We talked and talked about it together, and she eventually agreed to living in the Berry Brow/Newsome area of Huddersfield providing that the house we purchased was a new or fairly new one in a nice position in the area. We looked at possibilities throughout the Berry Brow area, including a relatively new housing site in Taylor Hill.

The site was being developed by Jack Brook Builders Ltd, a local company based at Thirstin Mills on the outskirts of Honley, a much larger village between Huddersfield and Holmfirth. They were known as a very reputable building concern throughout the area and almost all of their properties were built in natural stone rather than brickwork. The site we were looking at was called Bankfield Park and consisted of a number of three- and four-bed detached houses and two- and three-bed detached bungalows and dormer bungalows. The properties had only been built in small numbers at a time and were basically being built to order. I had seen a three-bed detached dormer bungalow being built which was basically just a shell and was apparently awaiting a buyer prior to being completed. The outer walls and roof were in situ, and the floor and ceiling joists were in place. The rest of the building was awaiting a buyer's preferred layout in respect of the rooms, kitchen and bathroom fixtures and fittings, etc.

I took Heather to see it one evening, and after seeing it and discussing the possibilities of the internal aspects, we both became quite excited about things.

The ground-floor design was originally to have a large lounge running the length of the building at the front, some 22" x 12" with a large bay window; the kitchen was at the rear left-hand side; a bathroom was in the middle; and bedroom three was at the rear right, with the main and second bedrooms on the first floor. It didn't take us long at all to change the design around more to our liking. We decided to leave the lounge and kitchen as designed but change the bathroom into a dining room and bedroom three into the bathroom. The staircase to the first floor would then be situated in the dining room, which would be open plan. Originally the staircase would have been in a corridor separating the original bathroom. The first-floor bedrooms would remain unaltered.

Much better!

With me working for A W Lumb & Co Ltd it was also advantageous to purchase the bathroom suite, kitchen fixtures and appliances through the company rather than Jack Brook Builders. As employees were allowed to purchase through the company at product cost plus five per cent, it represented quite a large saving. Needless to say, this is what we did.

Our first step after deciding that this was the house for us, was of course trying to arrange a mortgage in order to buy it. This we did and fortunately without problem through the Halifax Building Society, with whom I had been saving with for a few years. The cost of the house, after various amendments due to us altering the design and supplying various fixtures ourselves, was the princely sum of £13,383.28. We duly agreed to buy the property with Jack Brook Builders and arranged for Lumb's solicitors, Eaton Smith & Downey, to act upon our behalf in respect of the legalities required during the purchasing process. The solicitor to be dealing with the purchase on our behalf was Malcolm Tracey, who, I am delighted to say, continued to represent us whenever needed until his retirement in 2010.

We agreed to the purchase in November 1977 and moved into it on our wedding day of 22nd April 1978.

A copy of the invoice from Eaton Smith & Downey contains the details of the purchase of our new home at Bankfield Park Avenue, Taylor Hill, Huddersfield (see plates section figure 31).

Our wedding day was set for Saturday 22nd April 1978 and the ceremony to be held at St Mary's Church, Horbury Junction, at 11.00am. A few days prior to the wedding ceremony we attended the usual rehearsal at the church. When we entered the church that evening, we were both surprised and somewhat shocked to find that the interior of the church was being redecorated. Dust sheets, ladders, cans of paint and decorators' tools seemed to be everywhere we looked, and we were getting married two days later! The reverend apologised for the state the church was in and went on to assure us that the ceremony would not be affected much, if at all, as the decorators would be tidying the affected areas prior to the wedding ceremony.

Saturday arrived, and the ceremony went ahead as planned, and the decorator's equipment, whilst mostly still there, did not interfere with or affect our matrimonial ceremony. Before and after the ceremony the usual photographs were taken, some inside the church, as Heather and I were walking out hand in hand, but mostly outside of the church, along with our parents and guests.

The reception was held at the Shepherds Arms, Cluntergate, Horbury, and was attended by the majority of our wedding guests. Heather's parents, Pat and John, had arranged for a magnificent buffet lunch, and everyone tucked in and seemed to thoroughly enjoy themselves. Following the buffet and usual speeches, Heather and I drove to our newly awaiting house at Taylor Hill, dropped off presents that we had been given by various guests, changed out of our wedding attire and duly set off on our honeymoon, which was to be spent in Appleby, North Yorkshire.

I had never been to Appleby before but found it to be very pleasant and situated in a wonderful area with lots of open countryside all around. We thoroughly enjoyed our few days there before returning to our new house with excitement in abundance, as we were about to start our new lives together at number 42.

Whilst the inside of the house was all brand new, decorated and furnished to our liking, the garden areas outside needed a lot of hard work to make them actually look like gardens both front, side and rear. Over the next few weeks (and months), we set to, eventually turning all to our liking. The front and side garden areas took preference, and we found that the earth contained quite a depth of clay before soil was struck. We dug out as much as we could and replaced it with top soil that we acquired from another area of the site. This was done during the spring bank holiday period during May, and the weather was quite hot and sunny. We found it hard work, and with the sun beating down upon us most of the days, we suffered from sunburned skin on our arms and backs, which made it very uncomfortable when retiring for the night. After preparing the ground we purchased a suitable amount of ready to lay grass and – hey presto – the front and side gardens were looking good. A few plants here and there and a young rowan tree finished things off, and our hard work was considered very well worthwhile. We both felt very proud of ourselves.

We decided to give the house a name and Heather chose to call it simply "Rowan" after the tree we had planted. A little later, I found a suitable piece of slate, etched the name on it, painted the etching gold and fixed it to the house stonework at the side of the garage door. Another piece of slate was fitted to the fence at the top of the steps with the number 42 on it at the same time. Believe it or not – they are STILL there, exactly as they were in 1978, over forty years later.

The next step was, of course, the rear garden, which took quite a bit longer to complete as it was quite sloping from front to back, with the back being some ten feet higher than the front, which was the same level as the rear of the house. We decided to terrace the slope with steps built in the middle of the terraces leading up to a flat area of lawn at the top. The terraces on either side of the steps comprised of three terraces each side, supported by shallow dry stone walling. To finish things off various plants were bought and put in place. Again, we obtained ready-to-lay grass for the lawn area at the top, but this took us much longer than the front and side areas to complete. We also fitted a six-foot-high panelled fence across the rear with small conifers down the sides of the lawn area. When that was finished, I built a small barbeque area on the rear patio, which was laid by the builders after they had completed the construction of the house. Our house was now virtually complete with nice gardens to enjoy.

The first winter there turned out to be very cold. So much so that the net curtains over the window in the bathroom actually froze overnight to the glass on a number of occasions. Now when we bought the property, we did not have central heating installed as we could not really afford it at the time. The only heating installed was a gas fire in the lounge. The kitchen was always quite warm as the oven and hob were in constant use. During the Christmas holidays that first winter, I borrowed two "space heaters" from work in order to help keep the house, and ourselves, of course, warm.

Needless to say, we had a gas central heating system installed long before our next winter arrived!

For our second Christmas in the house we had invited my mum, dad and grandma to Christmas Day lunch. Heather had everything organised and was raring to go come Christmas morning and duly set to. The vegetables were prepared, the turkey ready to go into the oven and we virtually only had the table to set and we were ready for lunch. Into the oven went the turkey and we were away. Or at least so we thought. After about an hour we heard a loud "bang" coming from the kitchen and to our horror, we found that the oven had apparently exploded. Bang went the Christmas dinner, along with the oven! We had nothing in which to carry on cooking with, apart from the hob, and you can't cook roast turkey on one of those. Horror of horrors!

I can't remember how it came about, but our next-door neighbours Christine and Nigel Martin came to our rescue. They had arranged to go out to family for their Christmas lunch and insisted that we use their oven in which to cook the turkey and roast potatoes. Our bacon was saved, so to speak, and thanks to them, in the end all went well. It turned out that our double oven had not expired at all, but the wiring used during the installation was not of the correct size. It was far too small to cope with the power required by the oven when working at full or near full capacity. Oh dear, Heather's father, John, had installed it for us and he has been reminded of that day on many occasions since.

Not long after we married, we had an addition to the family – wrong! We had decided to buy a puppy. We had both come from dog-loving families and it seemed a natural thing to do. Heather looked at what pups might be available in the area and, after considering various possibilities, opted for a Cavalier King Charles Spaniel that had just been born to a family in Goole, North Humberside. Heather and her mother arranged to visit the family, look at the pups available and decided almost immediately upon a tri-coloured bitch. Shortly afterwards we were a family of three: me, Heather and Lisa.

One Saturday afternoon about a year later, I was sat in the lounge at home waiting for Heather to return from a shopping trip with her mother. I heard Heather's car pull up outside and her walk up the steps at the front of the house. The front door opened and in trotted Lisa, who went straight past the lounge door, which was open, through the dining area and into the kitchen. I then thought that I had suddenly seen something else, but I wasn't sure. In walked Heather, who bent down just outside the lounge door and ushered through a small puppy. Another Cavalier King Charles Spaniel, this time a Blenheim in colour. What a surprise. Totally unbeknown to me the puppy had been obtained from a family in Dewsbury as a friend for Lisa and was to be called Sadanka (later to be nicknamed Siddy). Although I was surprised at her appearance, it was a pleasant surprise. We were now a family of four. Lisa and Sadanka became good friends from the start, not only with us but themselves also and were virtually inseparable. Most of the time wherever one went the other followed, and they often played together as well. Whilst Lisa was quite a fussy eater, Sadanka would eat almost anything in sight, including Lisa's food if she got the chance. Sometimes I referred to her as Hoover because she ate like a vacuum cleaner – almost everything.

When we first married, we decided not to try to have children until we had become reasonably financially "settled", therefore being in a position to support them in the way we wanted to. Occasionally, Heather's aunty Iris would comment to other family members as to whether there might be something wrong in the lack of an announcement that Heather was expecting. There was nothing wrong whatsoever; we were both concentrating on our wish to have things in financial order before doing so.

During 1984 we decided that the time was right to try and start a family, and our first child, a daughter whom we named Laura, was born on 17th August 1985. Heather's pregnancy went very well throughout her term, and very few, if any, complications were experienced. The nine months seemed to pass quite quickly, and one Friday morning, 16th August at around 6.00am, I found myself driving Heather to Huddersfield Royal Infirmary. She was in the early stages of labour. We had contacted the hospital before leaving the house and they were expecting our arrival.

The arrival of our daughter Laura was not quite as organised and punctual as our arrival at the hospital that morning. Heather was taken to a maternity ward, with me following closely behind and allotted a bed in a private room. The time was still not long after 6.00am and the next few hours turned out to be the most excruciating hours that Heather had ever or was indeed ever likely to experience again in her lifetime. As the contractions came and went, the pain that Heather was experiencing was getting worse and worse. For hour after hour it went on and on. I was there almost all of the time, only excusing myself for the occasional toilet break. Heather found that when she wanted to relieve herself in that way, she could not go. Eventually she wanted to go so badly and still couldn't, that the nurses decided to insert a tube inside her and relief was finally at hand - with me occasionally holding the bottle.

The time went on and on. They say that time waits for no man. Time waits for no woman either, as we found out that day. Or, to be truthful, the day after!

At 3.17am on Saturday 17th August 1985, after around twenty-one hours in labour, Laura was born, coming into the world at 9lb 2oz. Heather had to endure a small amount of surgery during the delivery, as Laura was such a healthy-sized baby. I have often heard that mothers "forget" about the pain(s) of giving birth to their child once the delivery is completed, and Heather, although somewhat exhausted, seemed to be no exception.

I stayed with them both for about thirty to forty minutes before the nurses suggested that Heather should be allowed to rest following the birth, along with Laura, of course, and I duly made my way home. I immediately telephoned Heather's mother and father, and mine as well, of course, to give them the good news. I then retired to bed after setting my alarm for 8.00am. I had planned to go to both Heather's parents and mine that morning to tell them more. I had also taken a couple of photographs of them both on my Polaroid to show them. Just after getting up that morning, on the spur of the moment I decided to ring my Uncle John, who lived near Boston, Massachusetts, with the news. He asked me to give his congratulations to Heather and his love to Laura before asking me what time Laura had been born. When I replied 3.17am he immediately informed me that it was 3.17am at that very moment in Boston! Can you believe that? Perfectly true, I assure you!

After showering, shaving and dressing, I then telephoned my brothers, Stephen and Glyn, with the news. Shortly afterwards I went to see my parents and let them know more about Heather, Laura and the birth. I did not go into the detail much, except to tell them about the twenty-one-hour trying time that Heather had experienced. Following that it was a twenty-minute drive to Horbury to see Heather's parents, Pat and John. Upon arrival there I was in for something of a shock. In the kitchen area were Pat and John, with another gentleman who was apparently from the electricity board. He was demanding payment for a bill that had been unpaid and told them that if payment was not given to him, they would be cut off there and then. Pat and John had no cash in the house, and whilst they could pay by means of a card, they were told that would not be possible. Pat was obviously getting distressed, so I asked the man if he could accept payment from me by cheque. The answer was affirmative, the problem was solved and away he went.

I then told them the story of the day and night before, showed them the couple of photographs that I had taken after the birth, and that afternoon they visited Heather and Laura at Huddersfield Royal.

Both Heather and I were extremely touched by the number of congratulatory flowers, bouquets and presents that were afforded to all three of us, but Heather in particular, from family, friends and works colleagues alike. It is still gratifying to think back to that time and remember those things.

Heather remained in hospital for a couple of days or so before returning with our daughter to her new home and family life began in earnest – there were now five of us!

The next few months were both very exciting and occasionally tiring for both of us. I was very busy at work during the day, and Heather even busier looking after Laura, Lisa and Sadanka. Heather would take them all to her parents' house by car quite often during the day but was always back at home before I arrived from work. Evenings were always busy for both of us. Besides meals for us all, bath time for Laura, walks for the dogs and lots of other things needing to be done in between, the evenings went very quickly, as it must do and have done for all new parents.

Laura was not very good at going to sleep in the cot, which we had put in what was now Laura's bedroom, and cried and cried when left alone almost every night. We took it in turns to hold her and comfort her until she went to sleep in our arms before placing her as gently as we could into her cot. The number of times she woke up again almost immediately after she had been laid down was incredible. This went on for what seemed like months, but she gradually settled down to accepting what we considered to be normal.

Heather was now a full-time mother (to three) and housewife, and whilst I was aware that she missed working at Eurocopy, she never complained about anything and just got on with it all. When Laura was a few weeks old, Heather and her mother, who had seen a special offer advertised, took Laura on her first holiday. The three of them jetted off to Menorca for a week for £99 each with Laura free, leaving John and me to fend for ourselves. On their return telling us of what a good time they all had had, of course.

In July of 1986, of course, I lost my job at A W Lumb & Co Ltd, which, besides being somewhat of a bombshell, caused a prospective financial problem for us. A year or so earlier we had bought Heather a new car, a Skoda Rapid, on a hire purchase agreement. As long as I could obtain another job fairly quickly that was unlikely to cause too much of a problem. With my background and reputation in the area we didn't think that it would be a problem in doing so. It turned out that I would not secure another position until December, and by that time funds were running low. The monthly mortgage payments had to be met, the monthly hire purchase paid for and of course our living costs, which were not inconsiderable. As mentioned previously, I resigned from that job very quickly due to the reasons mentioned. Whilst I commenced the next one almost immediately, I took an extremely large reduction in salary, around £5,000.00 per annum, so something had to give. The only thing, really, was that the Skoda had to go.

Now this caused quite a large upset, not so much so with Heather, but with her mother, who really let fly with both barrels. She would not accept the fact that we could not afford everything at that time and that something had to give. Most unfortunately, even though I was as upset about having to make that decision, it was the only one we could really make to keep things going for us as a family. We managed without the Skoda for a few months until I had another opportunity, which came out of the blue in 1987 with Cooper Clarke Ltd giving me a much better salary and conditions. We were soon able to buy Heather another car, again a Skoda Rapid, but this time an almost new one and paid for rather than on hire purchase. Things were getting back to "normal".

During 1987 Heather became pregnant for the second time and her baby was due to be born in February 1988. Because of the problems giving birth to Laura in 1985, it was suggested by the maternity staff that Heather might consider having a caesarean section rather than a natural delivery. After a short deliberation this is what Heather decided upon and I fully supported her decision. The pregnancy went without concern, and on 22nd February our second daughter, Nicola, was born, weighing in at 8lb 3oz, another addition to our family which now became six. I was now well outnumbered, with five females to one of me!

Over the next few months Laura, who was now into her third year, was showing love and caring for her little sister, which was really nice for us both to witness. Lisa and Sadanka were very friendly with them both as well, of course. In fact, thinking back to when they were both newborn babies, Lisa and Sadanka showed real interest and obvious love with them both at all times. I cannot think of a time that they didn't.

In May 1988, Heather suggested that we might move to a new house into something a little bigger now there were six of us, to which I agreed. If we moved into a three-bedroom property, the girls could have a separate bedroom each, which would be better for them growing up, of course. With me working sometimes five days a week, and most Saturday mornings, Heather and occasionally her mother started house hunting. Now, I had always known that Heather would like to live in the Wakefield area, which was much closer to her heart than Huddersfield, so I was not surprised when a house in Lupset Park was mentioned as a possibility. With us having lived for the last eight years in my preferred location, I had no real objection in a possible move to Wakefield, subject to us both being totally happy with the chosen property, and with that area being much closer to where I worked, it also made sense.

An initial appointment to view was arranged and Heather went with her mother and the girls to look around it. She was very keen on it from the outset and quite naturally I agreed to accompany her for my first viewing of it a few days later. I also found the property to my liking, and after discussing things together, without involvement from her mother, we decided to put in an offer with the agent, which was of course subject to us selling our property. The property concerned was a three-bedroom detached house with a garage at the rear accessed via a driveway at the side and parking for at least a further three vehicles. In addition to the front garden there was a quite large rear garden, which backed on to the local municipal golf course. There were other detached houses at both sides and a mixture of detached and semi-detached houses across the road at the front. The address being Cleveland Grove, Lupset Park, Wakefield, and was currently owned by a Mrs Lawton, a widow, who was looking to downsize for obvious reasons.

Our offer was accepted, and we duly put our house on the market. This exercise was done entirely by Heather, who arranged for an advertisement to be placed in *The Huddersfield Examiner*. We had decided not to use an agent initially and the advert was therefore a private sale. The housing edition came out each Thursday evening and the printed editions were usually available for sale from 4.00pm at the various news stands in the town centre and delivered to the many newsagents shortly after.

At exactly 4.00pm that day the telephone rang, to be answered by Heather. It was a gentleman called George who worked for *The Examiner*, and he told Heather that he had seen the advert earlier in the day and that he wanted to buy the house. He informed Heather that he had to wait until the edition had been put on sale before he could put in an offer. This he was duly doing now, and his official offer was £42,000.00 – the asking price! The house was sold – a record, perhaps?

On 25th May 1988 we received a letter from the Halifax Building Society informing us that our application for a mortgage on the new property had been accepted, which also contained a copy of the house buyer report and valuation that was necessary. In early August we were actually moving into our new (to us) house at Cleveland Grove. It had taken less than three months from deciding to move to actually moving into the new house. We couldn't believe it.

The new property didn't need much doing to it apart from a really good clean and replacing all of the carpets, which did not take long to complete. Laura and Nicola now had their own separate bedrooms, Nicola's at the rear of the house next to our bedroom, both overlooking the rear garden, and Laura's at the front of the house overlooking the front garden. Lisa and Sadanka both settled in immediately, and our new adventure had begun.

The rear garden comprised of a vegetable-growing area rear right, a greenhouse (which was in some disrepair), two apple trees near the middle of the lawn areas, a fence across the rear and about ten quite large conifers down the whole of the left-hand side. These effectively separated our garden from next-door's garden. However, there was also a panelled fence behind the conifers. It wasn't all that long after we had moved in that we decided the conifers had to go. The earth all around them was so dry that it was more like dust than soil, and nothing would grow between them and obviously hadn't done for quite some time.

The front garden was also lined by a number of conifers, but the only thing we did with them was to give them a really good pruning. We also re-laid the flagstones which made up the driveway to the house, as they were quite uneven. The driveway was long enough and fairly wide nearer the house, and it was quite easy to park at least three cars there. The garage was at the rear of the property and accessed by car at the right-hand side beyond the driveway. The garage was not in the best of condition and I can't remember us ever using it for our vehicles. It was only used for storing gardening tools and the like.

We soon settled in and made it into our own home.

At this time, I was working for Cooper Clarke Group in the Hunslet area of Leeds, so it was quite a bit closer for me to get to work and back. The time saving was about twenty minutes each way. This was quite a considerable saving in both time and petrol, of course. We had only been there a few months when I was suddenly made redundant and I found myself out of work again. This was obviously a shock to us all, but having been through a similar situation previously, I wasn't as upset about it as I was on that occasion. I was, however, obviously upset about it, not to say surprised, and it was something that I hadn't thought possible as the division I was running seemed to be doing pretty well at the time.

I needn't have worried about it too much, as I was back in a new job within a week or so, this time working from home as area representative for Samson Lintels Ltd. My new office was soon to be established at our new house and things in general started to be on the up, so to speak. It was shortly after this that Heather had been considering going back to work herself, but only part time. Vacancies had arisen for telephone sales operatives at Empire Stores Ltd, a major mail order catalogue company based at Lupset, for two or three evenings each week for Friday, Saturday or Sunday evenings.

Heather applied and was soon working Saturday and Sunday evenings on a regular basis, along with the occasional Friday.

It turned out to be a good arrangement for us all. It gave Heather something different to do, me the opportunity to spend bonding time with Laura and Nicola, and additionally, some extra money coming into the household. It turned out to be good for us all. Heather would leave for work at around 4.30pm each evening, return around 10pm and I would generally have a meal ready for her return. The girls would have been in bed and asleep for some time, of course. Friday nights became something of a treat for us all. Heather and I would have a chilli pizza (with extra topping) and thin-cut French fries from the local Italian takeaway in Horbury, washed down by a bottle of red. Laura and Nicola usually had chicken nuggets and fries, but with a soft drink, of course. We had this virtually every Friday night and we really did look forward to it.

In late 1991 Heather and I decided to have the house altered and extended somewhat. Plans had been passed for the removal and demolition of the existing unused chimney at the side of the house and demolition of the garage at the rear. At the right-hand side of the house, a new garage and new kitchen, complete with utility area and a new sun lounge with archway access to the new kitchen across the rear. What was originally the kitchen would become the dining room. We had given the go-ahead to a builder that I had known from my days at A W Lumb & Co Ltd, David North (D M North Builder & Property Developer), based in Ossett, who had quoted a price in the region of £15,000 for the whole job.

As you will recall, the week before work was due to start on the house, Michael Miles, the general manager at Samson, had requested myself and the other sales representatives to help out with the stocktaking at the Samson premises in Gloucester. Samson Lintels had been sold to Catnic Components Ltd.

Well, I returned home that evening and we discussed the whole happening in more detail over our usual Friday night takeaway. On the Monday morning David North and his colleagues arrived as planned and the works commenced. It took quite a few weeks to complete, but when it was completed, we were absolutely "over the moon" with it. David and his colleagues did us proud, and we got exactly what we wanted, if not a little more.

The following year we all went on holiday to Menorca for a couple of weeks. This brought a few memories back to Heather, but it was a first for Nicola and me, and Laura was too young to remember that she had been there previously, of course. We hired a car and went all over the island. The weather was brilliant, and we all had an excellent time. I still remember that one day we went on a coach trip from the hotel to the main town of Mahon. There we visited a leather shop selling many different items manufactured in a very soft feel of leather. One such product being leather jackets, soft supple leather, lovely styling and finish – but what a price, very expensive – but advertised as being worn by Jasper Carrot the comedian. The prices weren't funny, though!

Most unfortunately, it was whilst living here, that first Sadanka passed away and not long afterwards so did Lisa. We had lost two very good friends that were very close to our hearts. A little while later we added another Cavalier King Charles Spaniel to our family, Sophie, again a Blenheim. A few months later, in 1995, I left Samson and joined Selflock, as previously mentioned, but the move did not turn out as originally planned or indeed expected.

The time seemed to pass very quickly. Laura had been at school for a few years and Nicola for about three, when towards the end of January, Selflock made me redundant, and the start for another form of employment began. We had said that if I ever were made redundant for a third time, we would look seriously about becoming self-employed. Well, here it was, number three. The search was about to begin, but in a different way. The search was on for our own business.

I think it was Heather's mother, Pat, that showed Heather an advertisement for a business that was on the market in a business for sale publication, *Daltons Weekly*. The business was a residential hotel, The Bossiney House Hotel, but was situated some 340 miles away in a village called Tintagel. Heather and I looked at the details, which were somewhat limited, but after talking and thinking about it we decided to arrange to view it through the business agents, Robert Barry & Co, based in Plymouth. We arranged to visit the hotel on 3rd February 1996, so we certainly weren't letting the grass grow under our feet.

Following our original viewing we were given an advertising recording (VHS) of the hotel and area by the owners, which we showed to Laura, Nicola and Heather's parents upon our return that night. We travelled down and back the same day – a long drive – but there were two of us doing the driving. A few days later we all went to view it, but this time hired a seven-seat vehicle in which to travel. Needless to say, after doing a lot of homework on it we decided to "give it a go".

We set to and put the wheels in motion. We made an offer for the hotel, which was accepted. We applied for the funding for the purchase of the hotel and various other things that were going to be required. The bank concerned, The Bank of Scotland, required us to submit a business plan, inform them of our insurers, our general bankers and of the dates that we were working towards. Our house was put on the market and a buyer obtained, one or two insurance policies were cashed in, and Heather's parents agreed to join us in Tintagel, then put their house up for sale to assist us with the purchase – and we still found ourselves £15,000 short. My uncle John, who lived in the USA, came to the rescue, and all things eventually complied with, the business became ours and we were away. All we required then was the date of completion – 4th May 1996.

Chapter 6

New Horizons

THE MONTH STARTED off really well. Things couldn't have been much better if you had written a script.

Heather and I, along with our children Laura and Nicola, had succeeded in purchasing a hotel in Tintagel, North Cornwall – The Bossiney House Hotel. It was quite large, being a twenty-bedroom holiday hotel set in grounds of approximately 1.5 acres of mainly lawned gardens. Overlooking the North Cornwall coastline and the South West coastal path, the hotel was mainly frequented by the walking fraternity and enjoyed a quite large overseas agreement with a Germany-based company, Wikinger Reisen, who specialised in worldwide walking holidays.

Soon to join us – the following week, in fact – were Heather's parents, Pat and John Cannings, who had helped us financially to buy the business and had agreed to join us in Cornwall to work at the hotel with us, on a part-time basis. In reality they were joining us to semi-retire.

We were very pleased with ourselves and proud to be the new owners of such a large and prominent business and premises. In addition to the hotel, we had also purchased a three-bedroomed cottage and separate two-bedroomed flat as living accommodation, all of which were situated in the same grounds.

We arrived at the hotel on a Thursday evening in early May 1996, to find the hotel closed for business due to our impending takeover the following day. Our takeover was subject to the local magistrate's court at Bodmin granting us a temporary licence in respect of the hotel bar. The hearing for the licence transfer was due to take place the following morning, Friday 4th May 1996, at 10.00am.

When we arrived at the hotel on the Thursday evening we were met by the then current owners, Bob and Margaret Savage, along with their son David. Bob and Margaret were in partnership with Bob's brother Colin and his wife Sandra, who were already living at their new home in Treknow, a small village just outside Tintagel.

The first thing we did after being shown to our rooms for the night was to unload the Ford Galaxy that we had bought a couple of weeks earlier, in which we had travelled down from Yorkshire. Sophie, our Cavalier King Charles Spaniel, was first out, quickly followed by Flopsy the rabbit and then our pet goldfish, all of whom had survived the long journey, thankfully, surprisingly well.

Having been in the car for some seven hours, we were, as you would expect, quite hungry and very definitely thirsty. We were hoping that we would be able to eat at the hotel that evening, but as stated earlier, the hotel was completely closed pending our takeover the following day. Bob suggested that we eat at a local restaurant in Tintagel called The Riggs. After putting the luggage away in our rooms, we drove down to Tintagel for a very welcome meal.

I don't really know what we all expected of The Riggs, but I know that I fancied a nice large steak with all the trimmings.

When we arrived and looked at the menu, we found that the restaurant was really a snack-type establishment rather than what we were hoping for – a really nice restaurant! Little did I know what was about to come. In fact, little did any of us know what was about to come!

The following morning, Friday 4th May 1996, the four of us drove to the magistrate's court in Bodmin, in order to attend the hearing for our licence to sell alcohol through the hotel bar facilities. On our arrival, a local solicitor, who had been appointed by Eaton, Smith & Downey to represent us at the hearing, introduced himself, informed us of the requirements and necessity of the hearing, and shortly afterwards in we went.

I don't recall the solicitor's name and during the hearing he could not remember our names either, as he had to refer to his notes every time our names were required to be mentioned. He did not appear to be well informed or hadn't bothered to revise his notes on the matter in hand. Or was it perhaps a solicitor being a solicitor and acting out a role, as we sometimes see in films? Whatever it was, we were not at all impressed. Even less impressed a couple of weeks later when we received his charges from Eaton Smith, which were over six hundred pounds for about ten minutes' work. We did question the amount involved and expressed our feelings, but we still had to pay the invoice. Thankfully the licence was granted, our solicitors were informed and the business transfer was duly completed. We were now the official owners of The Bossiney House Hotel.

Upon our return to the hotel, Bob, Margaret, Heather and I took stock of all the consumables that were to be transferred to us, agreed the total price to pay and arranged to meet the following morning to complete the payments that were still outstanding between us. The following morning Bob, his brother Colin and I met in the hotel office and discussed the payments still to be made directly to them. In addition to the consumables we had to discuss and agree the advanced marketing costs incurred by them, along with one or two other things. The cost of the consumables was agreed upon immediately, as it was a straightforward transfer of goods. In respect of the forward marketing costs, advertising of the hotel in brochures, books and magazines, etc., it was unfortunately not quite as straightforward.

Two of the points they had stipulated with the sale were that the proposed new owners would be expected to stand the cost of forward advertising and the current owners would keep the advance booking deposit receipts. We were not prepared to accept this arrangement and had discussed this with our solicitor, Malcolm Tracey, a couple of days prior to taking the business over. Now, advance advertising in the tourism industry, more often than not, has to be arranged months in advance, in some brochures over a year in advance. In 1995 they had arranged to spend almost five thousand pounds in the various features and they were expecting us to pay this amount to them. They would also keep the monies received in respect of deposits for 1996.

They had also stipulated that the current owners (themselves) would be responsible for any expenses incurred during or following the transfer of the business to new owners that remained still to be paid for. The point I raised with them that morning was that if they were expecting to keep the deposits received, then they had to pay for the expenses of arranging the basics of it in the first place. Colin disagreed with my reasoning, but Bob agreed to it, and following them briefly discussing it together, we all agreed that they could keep the deposits received but had to stand the advertising costs already paid for by them. We agreed to pay for any outstanding advertising costs.

Another stipulation in the sale agreement was that none of the previous owners would either start up or purchase a similar sort of business to that being sold within a number of miles of the hotel. When we had been with Malcolm Tracey a couple of days before, Malcolm informed us that he had received a fax from Colin that morning, informing him that he was purchasing a bed and breakfast and trout farm business situated at Rocky Valley, which was only approximately half a mile away from the hotel. This was obviously contrary to the agreement, but we informed Malcolm that we would discuss it with Colin on completion and asked him to reply to the fax as such. We eventually agreed to allow the purchase, but not until after the advertising disagreement had been resolved to our satisfaction.

It was then down to the business of running something entirely new to us, as the only introduction we had had in the hospitality business was using hotels occasionally ourselves. Neither of us had actually worked in one. Our philosophy was quite simple and straightforward, though – run the hotel in the way that we would like it to be if we were to stay there ourselves. Do that and we shouldn't go too far adrift?

The most important thing for Heather and me was, of course, the girls. Heather had arranged for them both to attend Tintagel Primary School, which was situated about a mile from the hotel along Molesworth Street just outside the village of Tintagel itself. Heather or Pat would drive them there each morning and pick them up again after school had ended for the day. Thankfully they both seemed to settle in well and quickly made new friends.

A very important part of our business plan was to keep all the existing members of staff employed in the positions they currently had. A smooth transition was considered essential if we were to succeed. After all, the existing staff knew their own responsibilities better than we did at that time. All members of staff, without exception, agreed to stay with us, including Margaret and her sister Sue. There were no guests staying at the hotel that night, but our first two guests, an elderly couple of ladies, duly arrived the following day on a two-week stay.

Heather's parents, Pat and John, along with Lucy, their pet Dalmatian, were due to join us the following Tuesday.

On Sunday 6th May a group of people from America (CTS Group) arrived for a stay of five nights, as arranged with the previous owners, and we, along with the chef/cook Rose, had planned menus for their stays beforehand. Most unfortunately, what we hadn't been informed of was the fact that they were all vegetarians. We had planned a completely different set of menus and had to improvise very quickly. Our first lesson had been learned – enquire as to the guest's type of diet prior to them arriving! On the Tuesday they had arranged a coach trip for the full day and informed us that they would not require an evening meal that night. As we only had two other guests in at the time, we gave Rose and the waiting staff the night off, and knowing that Pat and John were due to arrive that evening, we had planned an easy evening for ourselves. Or so we thought.

At around 5pm the group's guide telephoned us to inform us that they were now coming back to the hotel early and would after all require evening meals. Panic stations: telephone Rose to come in urgently – she did: try to arrange waiting staff – unsuccessfully. Heather and Rose quickly planned and cooked evening meals for all and, would you believe it – I and the guests themselves waited on their own tables, helped to clear up and seemed to thoroughly enjoy their evenings "entertainment". Pat and John arrived during the meal and couldn't believe what was going on. We obviously didn't involve them in things, as they had just arrived after an eight-hour journey. What a start to our new life as hoteliers.

The following day all of our furniture arrived with Pickford's Removals, and Pat, John and Heather arranged all to be moved into the cottage and flats. Heather, Laura, Nicola, Sophie and me into the cottage; Pat, John and Lucy into the adjoining flat. Other than that, not a lot happened that week, and we were all probably thankful that it didn't. Our first week was something of a handful to say the least, but we were finding our way around.

One of the contracts that the previous owners had secured was providing the local rotary club with the venue for their regular meetings, which was normally held every second Tuesday. They would hold their meetings, followed by a cooked lunch in the hotel restaurant. Naturally a charge was made both for the venue and the meals involved, and the first meeting under our tenure was to be on Tuesday 14th May, which was only ten days after taking the hotel over from Bob and Colin. Bob was at hand prior to that first occasion and advised us as to what was expected and informed us as to the type of meals they had been providing over the preceding couple of years. We were all looking forward to our first venture into the unknown and had planned the meal and were ready for the day.

On the Monday, Heather and her parents went out for a time and I continued to do various things in and around the hotel. In the early afternoon I had been typing a letter to our insurance broker, Speake Medley Ltd, based in Rawdon, Leeds. They were the brokers for A W Lumb & Co Ltd, and I had known Derek Speake, the owner, for many years. They were now acting for Heather and me, and were very instrumental in giving us much-needed advice in our new venture. I typed the letter which was in response to a letter received by fax earlier in the day concerning household insurance for Pat and John, and duly sent it by fax to Derek. Shortly after this I remember feeling rather dizzy and I went outside for a bit of fresh air. That did not seem to do much for me and I returned inside still feeling the same. Shortly afterwards Heather returned, with her parents, of course, looked at me and asked if I was feeling all right. She suggested I should sit on the settee in the guests' lounge for a while, which I did.

I was still feeling somewhat groggy for a while and Heather decided to call the doctor's surgery in Tintagel. She obviously suspected that something was wrong with me. We hadn't even got around to registering with the doctor at that time, but within a few minutes a Dr Garrod arrived and, following an examination, suggested that I may have had a stroke. He advised that I should go for a lie down and if I was not feeling better overnight or worse during the night, then Heather should call for an ambulance. Heather decided that I should remain in a hotel bedroom rather than at the cottage, where there were stairs to climb. Room 9 in the hotel was situated on the ground floor and only a few yards from the lounge. I stayed there for the night, but during the evening the hotel was open, and guests were in and around, and of course Heather had to attend to her responsibilities as well as me. She came in to see me every few minutes in order to make sure I was getting no worse and retired for the night with me immediately when she could do so. Whilst I was in bed earlier during the evening I needed to go to the toilet, and when I got out of bed I collapsed on to the floor. My legs would not support me, and it was then that I really knew that something was wrong. I can't remember whether I told Heather of this or not at the time, but early next morning, around 6am, Heather called for an ambulance, and within a short while I was on the way to hospital.

When Heather made the call she was apparently asked which hospital she wished for me to be taken to. Not knowing which, Heather asked the operator for advice. She was told that Truro Hospital was available but that I would have to wait in a corridor until a bed was available. Derriford Hospital in Plymouth was further away but a bed was immediately available. Derriford was the choice made. The ambulance arrived not much later, and I was on my way, with Heather following in the Galaxy. Heather later told me that just outside Tintagel, at the top of a hill the ambulance pulled in and stopped. Thinking the worst, she pulled in behind and was astonished to be asked which hospital

I was to be taken to. He and the driver had been told Truro, but Heather had told them earlier that it was Derriford. They proceeded to Derriford!

On Tuesday 14th May 1996 I found myself on my way to hospital having had a stroke just eleven days after starting our new venture. What a bummer!

On arrival at the hospital, I was admitted to a mixed reception ward containing some six men and women and allocated a bed. Heather was with me, of course, and, along with a nurse, proceeded to make me as comfortable as possible. At this time I was virtually unable to stand up without support, never mind even walk. The nurse showed Heather where one or two things were situated around the ward, including the toilet. Now, as I was unable to pay a visit to the toilet, the toilet had to come to me in the form of a bed bottle. Being unable to stand up and support myself, never mind holding the bottle and aiming the required part of my anatomy in the required direction, Heather had to play the part of the nurse for a few hours. I had various examinations during the course of the day, along with medication, of course.

During this early period of my problem I was also partially paralysed down the right-hand side of my body and had some difficulty in speaking. We got through a very trying day for both of us and it was soon necessary for Heather to return home to the girls for the night, which she reluctantly did. I recall very little of what went on over the next few hours, but as you obviously now know, I survived this extremely traumatic time in my life. My thanks go out to the hospital staff and to Heather in particular.

The following morning Heather drove back to the hospital again, spending most of the day with me. This was, of course, the Tuesday of our first rotary club lunch, and Heather informed me that Bob Savage had offered to help Pat and John through the lunch, as Heather and I were very much preoccupied with much more important things. During the day I was transferred to a male-only ward, where I was to spend the next couple of weeks. I had more tests during the day and it became quite apparent to all that I had indeed suffered a stroke. Heather returned to our new home once again following another very trying day for her. I was still unable to feel the full effects of the problem due to the dizziness and, of course, the light drugs I had been given.

Wednesday arrived and Heather returned once again to be with me for a few hours. She told me that the rotary club lunch had gone quite well under the supervision of Bob Savage and that Dr Garrod, being a club member, had been there. She informed me that her mother had asked him about the consequences of the problem I had experienced, and he told her that the next forty-eight hours could be crucial as to whether I survived or not. Heather spent a few hours with me again before going back once again to be with the girls. Before she left I suggested that she spend a little more time with girls, as I was being looked after by the hospital staff, and the travelling each day, along with her concern about the girls, was not going to do her any good. If anything untoward was mentioned about my health, either I or the hospital staff would let her know immediately. I know that this would not have gone down well with her, but our concern had always been, and still is, with the girls, and now of course, with their children as well.

On the Friday, a new patient arrived in the ward and was allocated the next bed to me. He had also suffered a stroke – his was down his left-hand side, mine was the right-hand side – and we were to become quite good friends during our time here. His name was John Ayre, and he had a café in Launceston. Just after he arrived, lunch was being served in the ward to the patients. Now John, seeing the food being served to everyone, asked one of the nurses for some for himself. The nurse's reply was that he would be unable to be given anything to eat or drink until a doctor had checked that he was able to swallow anything safely and that this would be done shortly. This upset John and he became quite aggressive in the language that he was using. Obviously the nurses were quite used to this type of situation and were very calm and sympathetic with him. This seemed to make John even more upset, and he kept on and on about it, demanding that he be given a little something at least. Being in the next bed to him, I decided to try talking to him and told him that the nurses were only doing their job and had his health interests totally at heart. After all, what would happen to him if he couldn't swallow properly and ended up choking himself? This seemed to calm him down and in due course a doctor examined him and gave the all-clear.

He thoroughly enjoyed his evening meal!

Over the next few days we talked about all sorts of things. His business, his family, his past and mine, of course. John was quite able in his walking and was allowed to walk around the ward unassisted, whereas I, being very unsteady on my feet, was only allowed out of bed with assistance from a nurse. The downside for John was that he could not control his left arm very well and was regularly bumping into things with it. He was fortunate that he didn't injure himself, as some of the knocks his arm took were quite hard. During the first week I had been in bed almost continually and only had my pyjamas and dressing gown available to wear. Towards the end of the week the nurses asked Heather to bring me some daytime clothing to wear, which was a pleasant relief for me. After a few days I was given a wheelchair in which to sit rather than be in bed all the time, and John used to wheel me around the ward in it. I had been advised not to wheel myself due to the stroke.

We had been in the ward for almost two weeks when John was informed that in a few days' time, he would be transferred to the rehabilitation unit next to the hospital, which was called

"Rowans". I found that quite emotional, as you may recall that Heather and I had called our first house "Rowan". Hearing the news, I asked if I was due to be transferred as well, but was told that as I couldn't yet walk unaided it would not be possible. Now, each day we were given physiotherapy, which included attempting to walk both with and without walking aids, and I was determined that I would be able to walk unaided in order to also be transferred to "Rowans". After a day or two I managed to pass the requirement, only just, I might add, walking along a corridor unaided but with a nurse and John at either side of me – just in case I fell over! I didn't, and a couple of days later, immediately before the spring bank holiday of 1996, I was transferred to the rehabilitation unit "Rowans".

A couple of days before we were due to be transferred, John suggested that we might go to the hospital restaurant two floors below our ward, and each have a full English breakfast in celebration. A brilliant idea, we thought, as we had not enjoyed this British traditional cuisine whilst we had been there for the last couple of weeks or so. We asked the nurse in charge of our ward if it was okay to do so and she said yes, subject to a couple of conditions. I was to remain in my wheelchair, John had to push me in it, we had to use the lift and definitely not use the stairs under any circumstances. If we encountered any problems we were to contact her. Great – away we went, with John pushing with his right hand and his left one flailing loosely as usual, occasionally hitting a chair or door handle on the way to the lift.

In to the lift we went, down two floors, along the corridor and in to the restaurant. We had made it there without a problem. We both ordered a full English breakfast with extra toast, and went to a table and waited for our very much-awaited treat to arrive. A short while later the waitress arrived with our meals, placed them on the table in front of us and away we went. Or so we thought. We looked at each other and immediately started laughing like we hadn't laughed for weeks. As I mentioned earlier, John could only use his right hand and I could only use my left hand. Well, we were absolutely snookered – stumped. We had realised that we couldn't cut our sausages up, our bacon up or even butter our toast without making somewhat of a mess. Fortunately the waitress came to our rescue once again and thankfully did the necessary for us. We enjoyed the breakfast very much – with many thanks to the waitress for the help!

At Rowans I was allocated a bed in a ward set up for four people. Beside myself there was John Ayre, Peter Mills, who had had a second stroke, and another man called Lester. I don't recall his surname but he was a farmer, I think from Devon. With that weekend being spring bank holiday, quite a few of the patients were allowed to go home for the long weekend, and whilst John and Lester were allowed to, Peter and myself were not as we could not walk well enough to be considered safe to do so. The rehab unit was effectively very quiet that weekend, as most of the staff had also been given a few days off. Heather visited me each day, but we both understood that she had to be with the girls and, of course, the hotel for the busy weekend. I don't know how she managed to fit everything in, but she did and I was, and still am, very grateful. What she had to endure during this period of our lives is testament to her feelings and strength of character. Without her, who knows what might have happened. Her mother and father also helped during this time beyond the call of duty, both with the girls and the hotel.

Immediately after the spring bank holiday weekend, the rehab unit resumed full operation and I was asked to attend for an assessment in the physiotherapy department. I attended as requested and was introduced to a physiotherapist called Kate Fathers, who was to become my main contact throughout my rehabilitation. During our initial conversation I told her that I expected to be fully recovered by the end of the month (June) and consequently back at our new business. Kate asked me what gave me the impression that would happen and I replied that it was a state of mind over matter. Her polite reply was that we would work together with the end of the month as a carrot, but I had to do everything I could to adhere to the many exercises, requests and medications that would be forthcoming over next few weeks. She also advised me that the stroke I had endured was quite a bad one and that it was imperative that I did not try to overdo things. She also informed me that I was to be given a wheelchair to use at all times, and only to walk around when asked to do so by the physiotherapy or nursing staff.

My rehab had started under her watchful eye and I was given a basic timetable of the various happenings that would be ongoing for the foreseeable future. Breakfast would be served from 8.30am, lunch at 12.30pm and evening meal from 5.30pm in the communal dining room. Each morning at breakfast, all inpatients were given an individual form with their name, along with lunch and evening meal menus included, and all we had to do was tick our preferred choice and hand it back. I was also given a time to attend physiotherapy in the gymnasium area each morning, but a day in advance, as the times varied occasionally. Each afternoon I would attend the occupational therapy department, which specialised in hand, fingers, arms and body movements, in order for affected body parts to become more dexterous once again.

I must say at this stage that I don't recall turning down any menu offered throughout my three-month stay here. All lunch and evening menus contained a sandwich option if that was preferred for any reason. The standard of the food offered and served was extremely good at all times.

During mid June, Heather and I were asked to attend a short assessment with regards to the treatments I was to receive there, along with an approximation of the expected time to be spent in the unit. When Heather arrived she gently and discreetly informed me somewhat of a bombshell. It was concerning Roslyn and Brent Taylor, two of our best friends who were also godparents to our daughter Laura. Brent was also a prominent business colleague of some twenty years, being my main contact at I G Lintels Ltd, a major supplier to the builder's merchants that I had worked for previously. Roslyn had telephoned Heather with the devastating news that Brent had most unexpectedly died during a private operation for the fixing of a gastric band on 11th June. That was a tremendous shock to say the least. How Roslyn and their son Arron must have felt – I can't contemplate even now?

I don't recall the details of the assessment, as my thoughts and mind were in a completely different world.

Treatment continued at Rowans, and whilst my right arm, leg and foot were quite badly affected by the stroke, I felt that slight improvements were forthcoming, if rather slowly from my point of view. Kate did remind me from time to time that my condition was serious, but given time would improve, provided that I followed their treatment schedule.

Quite a few of the patients at Rowans were there for vastly different reasons, not only stroke victims. There were a couple of patients suffering from multiple sclerosis, a young lady called Becky suffering from severe depression, a man in his thirties called Glyn who had suffered a broken neck and was paralysed from his neck downwards, among others. John and I became quite good friends with Glyn and visited him in his room almost every day. He was most unfortunate to receive such a life-changing accident playing Rugby Union for his local club team. He was not a regular player, having retired a couple of years earlier, but continued to train and coach the team a little. One weekend he was asked to play for the team as they were short of players due to injuries. It was in this match that he received this horrendous, life-changing injury.

After John and I had been at Rowans for a while, we started to help the nursing staff during mealtimes by helping to feed some of the patients who could not really feed themselves without help. There were only a couple of nurses on duty during mealtimes, and with a dozen or so patients to assist, some patients were having to wait and their meals were going cold before they could be fed. We found this to be quite satisfying and were pleased to be of help to both the patients and, of course, the nurses. After all, we were all in it together.

I was gradually improving with my movements and in particular with my balance when walking. I was still using a wheelchair, except for when taking physiotherapy and occupational therapy, of course. Because of my improvement, I asked if it would be possible for me to return home each weekend as some other patients were allowed to do. The answer was yes, provided I used the wheelchair and did not overdo things, particularly walking. The hospital gave me the okay and Heather arranged to pick me up, along with the wheelchair, late each Friday afternoon and return me to Rowans on Sunday evening. This was just the tonic I felt I needed, especially as our main trade at the hotel, the Wikinger Reisen walking groups, were starting to arrive every twelve days through to September. Even though it was only for the weekends, I felt to be a part of the business for the first time since that fateful day in May.

Whilst I had been in Rowans, away from the business completely, I hadn't realised what had apparently been going on at the hotel. Heather had of course been spending time between seeing me, the girls and trying to attend to the hotel business which was completely new to us all. Not an easy task by any standards. It was a good job that her parents Pat and John had been there in more ways than one. However, it had become apparent to Heather that they were seemingly taking over the business. They did not seem interested in listening to how Heather wanted the business to be run but doing it their own way. I had not been near the hotel for obvious reasons and was unaware that even the hotel staff were somewhat unhappy about things. Heather was told that whilst she had informed members of staff one thing, her parents, particularly her mother, had told them to do things in a different way. This obviously caused concern and uncertainty with staff members, as they did not know who was running things!

One day, Heather heard from someone in the village that a member of staff had said that they were fed up of the situation, as Heather was instructing and saying one thing, and immediately her back was turned, her mother was changing that completely. This was obviously not on and Heather was forced to say something about it. By rightly doing so, this caused a lot of friction between Heather and both of her parents. Arguments became a regular part of the day and nights for some time to come. Most unfortunately, this affected both Laura and Nicola, who were totally innocent and unaware of what was causing the friction and seemingly endless arguments. As I was only at the hotel for a few hours at weekends, I was unaware of the daily situations.

Over the next few weeks things did not get much better and the arguments continued, as Heather informed me during her frequent visits to Rowans and of course my weekends at the hotel.

At the beginning of August, my younger brother Stephen suggested that he and his wife Carole could perhaps visit us and stay for a few days. His idea was that as I was virtually unable to write, we could purchase a computer, which would effectively enable us to complete the paperwork, which was necessary in the running of the business. He and my youngest brother Glyn, who was our accountant, would devise a spreadsheet enabling us to record the whole of our income and expenditure, compilation of restaurant menus, and all the other paperwork necessary. It would be much easier for me than trying write left-handed, not to mention much neater. It would also alleviate quite a lot of paperwork for Heather, who had her hands more than full with everything else that was or wasn't going on at the time.

Stephen and Carole duly arrived, and a couple of days later when I was at home for the weekend, we drove down to PC World in Plymouth. After looking at the systems available, Stephen, who had spent most of his working life in communications with Cable & Wireless, one of the world's largest communications companies, recommended that we choose a computer manufactured by Dell. After choosing a printer and a few other items, we returned to the hotel armed with the necessary armoury to attack the growing amount of paperwork, etc. Over the next few days he compiled detailed programmes for us to use in the various aspects required. This included a spreadsheet system in order to keep the daily, monthly and annual accounts correctly. The system was devised along with my youngest brother Glyn, and I still use that system to this day. Although the businesses have changed a little over the years, it has been an easy task to amend the business names and income and expenditure categories to suit. A few years later, Glyn also supplied us with a VAT calculation spreadsheet, which is also still in quarterly use as required by HMRC.

During that time I was still going back and forth from the rehabilitation unit to the hotel, and the situation between Heather and her parents was not getting any better. On occasions I was also drawn into it, but I was obviously on Heather's side. I don't recall the circumstances, but I was back from the rehab unit for the weekend when something occurred and I became very upset and annoyed. I was upstairs at the hotel doing something around rooms 14 and 15 at the time. Stephen and Carole were there at the time and I suddenly started to cry – yes, cry! I somewhat poured out my feelings to them and decided there and then that things had to change. Heather was under extreme pressure with everything that was going on and it was very definitely not her fault at all. At that very moment I decided to discharge myself from hospital and return full time to the business, even though deep down I knew that it was the wrong thing to do from a health point of view. I asked Stephen to drive me to the hospital that very afternoon to inform them of my decision and collect my belongings.

Being the weekend, staff at the rehab unit was minimal and the male nurse in charge was not one of the usual members of staff. When I informed him that I was there to discharge myself, he, in no uncertain terms, informed me that I was not allowed to do that. My reply was quite the opposite and I continued to pack my belongings, informing him that I was not a prisoner there and that there was nothing he could do to stop me. A few minutes later we were back in Stephen's car and starting the forty-odd-mile journey back to Tintagel.

The following morning, Monday, we received a telephone call from two of the physiotherapists at the unit, Kate, my usual physiotherapist, and Carol, the head of the occupational therapy department, who asked me the reasons for my decision. They seemed very understanding but stated that they thought it would be better for me to continue treatment at the rehab unit for a few weeks longer. I reiterated my reasons for not doing so and they then suggested something of a compromise. They asked if they could come to the hotel to assess the premises, in respect of my safety within the confines of the complex. They came later that week and made one or two suggestions regarding my safety in certain areas, a second handrail up the staircase in our living accommodation and taking extra care when bathing, etc.

They also suggested that I should continue to attend the rehab unit twice a week in order to receive physiotherapy treatment. A hospital outpatient voluntary vehicle service was available throughout Cornwall at a very small charge of £3.00 per return journey. We agreed to all the points made and accordingly I continued the treatment for the next few months. When that eventually came to an end, they arranged for a physiotherapist to treat me at home for around a further six months.

I was back at work, even though not doing the jobs that I had expected to be doing when we were initially planning everything. But at least I felt that I was contributing and that Heather had some support immediately at hand. Hopefully the extreme pressure that she had been under should be alleviated at least a little. It was – but not to the extent that it should have been. Pat and John were still very reluctant to change their ways.

Now please don't get me wrong. If it hadn't been for Pat and John's initial unexpected and absolutely necessary involvement, the whole venture may well have been a complete disaster. As you can probably visualise, the situation that occurred within the first ten days of our venture is probably one similar to a film writer writing a script for a possible disaster movie with virtually no holds barred. The husband hospitalised, the wife thrown in at the deep end, the children not knowing really what was going on, not knowing which way to turn or when, the parents/in laws having to learn how to "swim" without lessons and the staff not knowing who to respond to.

I fully well know that if it had not been for Pat and John, survival would have been very difficult.

However, I don't think that I or Heather, and possibly our daughters as well, will ever forget some of the things that went on, or indeed many of the things that were said, during the five years or so between our buying and selling of the hotel.

Our main customers at the hotel were annual visitors

from Wikinger Reisen, a well-known German company, who specialised in walking holidays throughout many countries of the world. The previous owners of the hotel had built up a relationship with them over the two years or so prior to our ownership, and we were very keen to continue and hopefully improve that relationship. Every year, Wikinger booked holidays for six and sometimes seven groups of people for a twelve-day period, comprising up to twenty-four guests plus a Wikinger tour guide. The hotel reserved fifteen rooms for each group, allocating the rooms depending upon the split of guests involved in each group. The bookings generally commenced late June through to early September each year. Consequently I "missed" the first group completely, but was there at least during the weekends during the most of July and August before discharging myself from rehab in late August.

The groups were booked in for dinner, bed and breakfast, and we organised their itinerary in advance for the duration of their stay. The daily itinerary for each group comprised of three daily excursions by coach to Lanhydrock House, The Lost Gardens of Heligan and St Michaels Mount, three escorted walks, one free day, and the remaining days for various walks under the guidance of the Wikinger tour guide that accompanied each of the groups. The escorted walks were led by our own guide, who was originally planned to be me, but due to my problem the reigns were taken over by Heather's father John. Now John has always had a specific type of humour and he immediately introduced himself to the members of the groups as "Sir John" and consequently he became known in this manner by all. So much so that future visiting members of the groups were asking who Sir John was, almost immediately they first arrived at the hotel. When I eventually returned towards the end of August, I had my own bit of fun regarding his new title by telling the groups that he was actually called "Serf John".

The groups were a very important part of our business, and we all became very close and friendly with them, treating them with respect and looking after them, as you would expect hoteliers to do with their guests. We also earned their respect, and even to this day, some of the guests that stayed with us at that time call in at our current business to say hello and enquire as to our health, etc. It is very satisfying for this to happen and it just goes to show that we must have done our job well.

In 1999 Wikinger approached us during the winter asking if we could accommodate a special group from 5th–12th June, in addition to their usual bookings, which had already been confirmed. Apparently a lady called Renate Bollwein had specifically requested that they arrange for a group of some twenty people to stay at Bossiney House for the duration upon a dinner, bed and breakfast basis, and for us to arrange a few days' itinerary for them. Additionally she had requested one of their regular tour guides, Klaus Freitag, to lead them. We knew Klaus very well, as he was a regular visitor to Bossiney from time to time with the Wikinger groups. Naturally we agreed to the booking and the week went extremely well and all enjoyed their stay with us. A caricature was drawn by one of the guests totally unbeknown by any of us until their final night with us, when it was presented to me (see plates section figure 39).

I feel that this sort of gesture just goes to show that doing one's best, and I mean everyone involved, is well worth doing. I did not, by the way, do any of the hotel's cooking, as mentioned in the above, but I did wait on and help with the washing up, etc., occasionally.

As I have mentioned already, some things that were apparent were simply not things that should be done in any type of business, but particularly in a service and hospitality business such as a hotel and/or restaurant. A couple of examples of this were directly related to John, Heather's father. On one such occasion, a guest by the name of Norman Walsh, a self-employed vibration engineer who was a regular visitor to the hotel whilst working at the Dairy Crest Cheese factory at Davidstowe, was having his evening meal in the restaurant and asked John for a half bottle of the house red wine to accompany his meal. John's immediate reply was that we didn't serve half bottles but he could have a full one. Norman declined the offer and John returned to his duties in the bar. A few minutes later John returned to Norman's table and put a cider bottle on it informing Norman that the bottle contained the equivalent of a half bottle of red which he had poured for him from a new full bottle. Now Norman did not tell me about this until after the restaurant had closed and we were in the process of tidying up from the evening activities.

When everyone had retired for the night and John and I were the only ones left, I brought the situation up with him and asked him what had gone on with Norman and his request for a half bottle of wine. His response was that he had served him with a half bottle in a rinsed-out cider bottle. I pointed out in no uncertain terms that to do something like this was definitely out of order in a number of ways. A rinsed-out cider bottle containing wine? Could that also be a health problem? What on earth would a guest think about that? Report us regarding health and safety issues? Would the guest return again? Why didn't he use a half carafe from behind the bar instead of a cider bottle of all things? Why didn't he at least suggest a full bottle to be consumed over two nights? John's reply was that if I wasn't happy about it I could do it myself in the ******* future and he stormed out, leaving me to finish off.

On another occasion he was waiting on and taking meal orders in the bar whilst I was working behind the bar. It was a particularly busy night as we had a Wikinger group in and quite a few non-residents in from the caravan site next door. John had been busy taking orders and passing them into the restaurant, when a member of the Wikinger group asked him a question. After a few minutes one of the non-residents interrupted John, who was now talking generally rather than answering a question. The man asked John if he was interested in taking their order or not, to which John answered rather abruptly that he was obviously talking to someone and that he would have to wait until he had finished. John could have easily excused himself from the conversation and returned to it within a couple of minutes.

Another situation that arose did not concern any guests but caused quite a lot of concern to John's wife Pat, Heather and myself. I don't recall how the situation arose in the first place, but Pat brought to our attention that John had been drinking quite a lot of whisky from behind the bar. In order to hide the fact from me perhaps noticing it, he had been replacing the whisky he had been drinking by pouring tap water into the bottles situated on the optics behind the bar. I hadn't noticed, but a situation of that sort could have been very serious had the weights and measures department been involved for any reason. John's health might also have been a major consideration had it continued. I did say shortly afterwards that if it was a case of him not wanting, or being unable, to pay for a whisky now and again, I didn't mind him having one or two occasionally as long as he did not replace it with water or overdo it.

During the first three years of owning the hotel we had more than our fair share of ups and downs, arguments, fallings out and disagreements with both Pat and John. It had become a regular happening for one and sometimes more of the above, to be occurring on a regular basis. At times we were expecting something to occur almost every time we saw them. It was also having a very bad effect on Laura and Nicola, as well as Heather and me. Quite often the girls would be upset and crying when

Heather returned to our living quarters after we had dealt with the evening's meals. Obviously this upset Heather quite a lot and was often due to something or other that Pat had either said or done.

During 1999 it became too much for Heather, and to a quite large effect me also, so we decided enough was enough. We contacted Robert Barry & Co in Plymouth, the chartered surveyors that we had purchased the hotel through, and arranged to put the hotel back up for sale with immediate effect. This was not something that we had decided upon without due thought and consideration, but unfortunately the overall situation demanded it. Heather in particular, the girls and I had had more than we should have had to take. Neither Pat nor John was happy about the decision we felt we were forced to make, but the hotel was duly put up for sale.

It didn't take Robert Barry & Co very long to achieve interested parties in the business, and before long a family, who were looking for a similar business in the area, became extremely interested. So much so that they offered, through Robert Barry & Co, the asking price, and the sale started to go through the usual procedures.

After a few weeks Heather and I were having second thoughts about selling and generally discussed the situation between ourselves. Pat and John were also concerned in a similar manner to us and after quite a lot of discussion between the four of us we decided on a different course of action. Pat and John informed us that they had decided to leave their accommodation within the hotel grounds and purchase a bungalow in nearby Tresparrett. In order to do this they demanded the immediate return of the £45,000 that they had lent us in 1996 in order to help us purchase the business. The amount was much more than we could afford to pay back outright, but a solution was not far away.

At the outset of our purchase in 1996 we borrowed £227,250 from the Bank of Scotland, which was to be repaid over a twenty-year loan facility. Heather and I had sold our house in Wakefield and cashed in a couple of insurance policies, and Pat and John loaned the £45,000. I had also assigned a low cost endowment mortgage policy to the bank that was now almost due for maturity. In order to return the money to Pat and John I arranged a further short-term loan with the bank of £20,000, of which £15,000 was to be transferred to Pat and John immediately, and instructed the bank to transfer a further £30,000 to them from the hotel current account.

Laura and Nicola were at the top of Heather's and my considerations, and we were both of the opinion that we should give things another go, particularly with them in mind. The arguments, fallouts, disagreements, etc., had to stop in order for things to become as we had originally intended. Heather and I were in charge of the way the business was to be operated and things had to change for the better without delay.

Pat and John informed us that they would like to continue working at the hotel and that by moving into their own home once again would hopefully enable them to relax and be back to being alright with us all.

We duly gave back word to Robert Barry & Co, explaining our reasoning, of course, and they informed the prospective purchasers accordingly. This decision did not come cheap. Because we had agreed to sell the business, a purchaser had been found at the agreed asking price and the paperwork had commenced, we were subject to a cancellation fee of £6,600.00. This fee could be deducted from any future commission charges that might become due to be paid to Robert Barry & Co should we decide to sell the business through them in the not too distant future.

For the next few months, things settled down somewhat and the business grew pretty much in line with our forecasts.

Unfortunately the situation with Pat and John did not last the course and it wasn't very long before we were back to the now familiar discourse within the business and family. In 2001 Heather and I decided once again to sell the business, as the stress caused by the constant fallings out and arguments was not considered worthwhile for any of us. Robert Barry & Co was re-appointed accordingly and the business was once again on the market.

It wasn't long before prospective buyers were found and following various visits to the hotel, telephone calls and information regarding the business accounts, etc., the deal was finalised. The new owners were new to the trade, as we were back in 1996, and a bit older than we were. They seemed very keen to commence their new existence and a date of 1st June 2001 was agreed for the sale to be completed. Our solicitor, Malcolm Tracey of Eaton, Smith, Marshall, Mills, set to work, and the sale was completed on the above date as planned at a selling price of £370,000, excluding the building and garden that we were now living in. Heather and I had been using Eaton, Smith since we agreed to buy our first house in 1977, prior to us getting married in April 1978, and I had known Malcolm since 1974 when I joined A.W. Lumb & Co Ltd.

A few months earlier, Heather and I had decided to separate one of the buildings within the hotel grounds, in order for it to become our home. Originally, the ground floor of this building was used as two hotel bedrooms and the first floor as accommodation for the then hotel owners Colin Savage and his wife and family, with Bob and Margaret Savage and family residing in a three-bedroom cottage attached to the hotel. We had used the buildings in the same way since we purchased it in 1996. There was also a considerable area of garden at the rear of the building, which we also separated and fenced off from the hotel rear garden area. We considered that this made the property an extremely desirable detached four bedroom (three with en-suite facilities), separate house bathroom, a large open-plan lounge and dining area along with separate kitchen. There was also an open area on the ground floor leading out into the rear garden that we had closed off and converted into a second reception room. At the front there was also a large double garage with plumbing for use as a washroom, etc., outside parking for a number of vehicles and a small lawned area. We had this property removed from the land registry details for the hotel and re-registered it in our own names as our residential accommodation.

After the sale of the hotel, we continued to reside in the property, which we had named “Westcote” (the three-bed cottage being “Southcote”), for about a year. During this time Heather mentioned on a number of occasions that she wasn’t very happy having to see the hotel from the house lounge and kitchen windows, and of course every time we left and returned to the house. She didn’t feel at all “at home” or relaxed having to live with it. Consequently in March 2002, Westcote was put on the market and we began looking for a new home. The house hadn’t been on the market long when a man called David Clark and his partner Ms Conrich, who were connected in some way with motor racing and based at Silverstone, the home of British motor racing, agreed to buy it. Unfortunately, the month before he and his partner were expecting the sale and purchase to go through, something most unexpected happened.

My mother had been in the Huddersfield Royal Infirmary for a few days and was expecting to be discharged, when my father was also admitted, with a stomach complaint. There being no-one at home to look after her, she was advised to stay in hospital for another day or so pending Dad’s discharge. Dad had only been in hospital for a couple of days when on Thursday 16th May 2002 we received a telephone call to inform us that he had passed away suddenly and unexpectedly. I told Heather that I was going to go straight to Huddersfield and she said that she would come with me. I said that she should stay at home looking after Laura and Nicola, but she wouldn't have it, ringing her mother and father and arranging for them to look after the girls for a few days.

We had a small argument about it at the time as I thought that Heather should be looking after the girls and not her mother and father, particularly after the "goings-on" with them only a few months beforehand. On reflection she was entirely right in insisting she accompany me during this time. The following day we duly made the six-hour or so journey to Huddersfield, staying at the Midgeley Lodge at Flockton, a small village four or five miles outside Huddersfield for the duration of our stay. We visited Mum in the hospital, where my youngest brother Glyn met us, along with his wife Yvonne. My younger brother Stephen and his wife Carole also joined us the next day.

Mum was taking the news extremely badly but was pleased to see us all there. We all tried to make her as comfortable about the situation as possible and she eventually seemed to be accepting it, although reluctantly. The four of us stayed in the accommodation we had booked for the next few days, with Glyn and Yvonne staying at their home on Bankfield Park, of course. Worse was to come, however.

On the Monday, Mum was not feeling at all well and the medical staff informed us that they were very concerned about her. On the Tuesday we were taking it in turns to be with Mum throughout the day, and on Tuesday night Stephen and Carole insisted that we all retired to our accommodation for the night and they would stay at the hospital with Mum. They rang us early on Wednesday morning 22nd May 2002 to inform us that Mum had just passed away. Both of our beloved parents had passed away within six days of each other.

The doctor who was present that morning informed us that he considered that Mum had passed away due to a broken heart.

Somewhat ironically, Mum and Dad were married on 15th May 1948 at St Paul's Church, Armitage Bridge, Huddersfield, and celebrated their golden wedding on 22nd May 1998 at Longley Park Golf Club, Huddersfield.

The month of May now has quite mixed feelings for me, as the following perhaps signifies.

May 15th 1948 – Mum and Dad married
May 22nd 1998 – Mum & Dad celebrated their golden wedding
May 4th 1996 – Heather and I purchased the Bossiney House Hotel
May 13th 1996 – I had my stroke
May 16th 2002 – Dad passed away
May 22nd 2002 – Mum passed away
May 10th 2019 – I had a total left hip replacement

A joint funeral was arranged, which took place on 31st May 2002, and their ashes were interred together at Hall Bower Cricket Club a couple of weeks later. Knowing how much they both loved the club, we felt that it was an appropriate resting place for them to remain together forever.

Shortly after we returned home, the house sale went through and we moved to our new home at Trewethen Barn, Tregatta, Tintagel, situated approximately half a mile away. The house had been converted from a barn a couple of years before and was totally different from anything else we had previously owned. It was situated on a plot of land covering about half an acre in size consisting of a mainly grassed area, with parking for four or five cars in addition to an integral garage. There were also two outbuildings, previously used as cow sheds, we think, but these were in need of extensive renovation and something we never got around to. With the grassed area being so large we decided to purchase a sit on motor mower, which was £1,000 very well spent and saved a lot of time as well as the energy required walking a standard motor mower around! The building itself comprised of three double bedrooms, a lounge, a dining room, a house bathroom and quite a large kitchen. We converted part of the garage, which was situated underneath the lounge area, into a study and small toilet. Peter Dyer, the local plumber, fitted a toilet area and new radiators, therefore making the new rooms much warmer when required. There was also a loft area, which was completely boarded out and accessed via a pull-down loft ladder. We lived here for around a year before deciding to move once again.

It was whilst we were living here that during 2003 our eldest daughter, Laura, met her now husband Daniel. They hadn't been going out together for very long when Laura informed us that she was pregnant. It wasn't only a shock to us; it must have been a shock to them as well, because after a few days Daniel went missing and no one, not even his mother and father, knew of his whereabouts. After a few days he returned, full of remorse and sorrow for his actions, and a few weeks later they decided to move in together and rented a flat in Trethevy, a small village just outside Tintagel on the B3263 Boscastle Road.

Towards the end of 2003 Heather and I decided to move from Tregatta and duly put the house up for sale. It wasn't very long after that we received an acceptable offer for the property, and in December of that year we were on the move again. We had seen a couple of properties for sale in Trethevy, believe it or not, and arranged to view them both. The first viewing was at a property called Westaway, a four-bedroom detached dormer bungalow overlooking the Atlantic Ocean situated approximately 400–500 yards away. The property was about six years old and had been built by Steve Wood, a local builder who lived next door in an identical bungalow that he had also built. We viewed the property, and both Heather and I were very impressed with it.

After the viewing, as we were leaving, Steve's wife June was mowing the lawn at the front of their house. I attracted her attention and she duly stopped and came over to the low wall adjoining the properties. Jokingly I told her that she needn't mow the lawn for our sake, as we had arranged to view their property the following morning and we had obviously seen the lawn in its more natural state. She laughed thinking that we were joking, but we weren't – we had arranged a viewing of it! This property was called Trebartha and had an identical view over the ocean. The bungalow itself was identical to next door on the inside except for the internal doors, frames and skirting boards. In Westaway the owners had painted them all white, whereas originally they were all stained mahogany as they were in Trebartha. Both Heather and I very much preferred the stained mahogany to the painted ones. Following the viewing we made Steve and June an offer, which was accepted. Exchange dates were arranged on both properties, and a few weeks later, on 21st December 2003, we moved in.

It was only a few weeks after we moved in to Trebartha that Laura gave birth to her first baby. On 17th March 2004 Sophie arrived – our first grandchild. With Laura, Daniel and Sophie living only a couple of hundred yards away, it was very easy to keep in touch with and visit them. There were about seven flats in the building and most unfortunately all were in need of refurbishment. The landlord seemed very reluctant to do anything for the tenants and they had to deal with the agents rather than the landlord. Their flat was very draughty, and when it rained the window and doorframes leaked. They were forever drying up and trying to stop the draughts, and it wasn't very long before they decided to move out. Their next 'port of call' was a rental in Boscastle, but after they had decorated and made the house to their liking, they once again discovered damp – this time not the window frames, etc., but rising damp. Time for them to move yet again. Over the years they must have moved at least eight times before finally buying their present four-bedroom detached house in December 2019 situated at Valley Truckle on the outskirts of Camelford. Rather than renting, they are buying the property, having obtained a mortgage. They are now a family of five, with Chloe being born on 26th January 2008 and Isaac, the most recent addition to the family, born on 17th December 2019.

Not long after they moved into the house in Boscastle, there was a catastrophe in the village. On 16th August 2004 we experienced an extremely bad cloud burst for a period of time. Heather and I, along with two friends, Sylvia and Laurie Tall, whom we had befriended through our hotel days, went for a lunch at a restaurant in Wadebridge. It was a beautiful day weather-wise, and it was so warm that we had been sat outside eating our meals in shirt sleeves. On the way back home to Trethevy the skies became very dark and it started raining extremely heavily. Heather was driving, and as we were approaching Camelford Station on the B3262 the road had become some five or six inches deep with fast-flowing rainwater. Normally we would have turned left opposite the cycle museum and travelled on the B3263 towards Tintagel. Due to the extremely poor driving conditions we decided to continue on the B3262 directly towards Boscastle as it was a more straightforward road for driving along. Heather was very attentive and drove steadily through all the rainwater, and we arrived safely at our house. We didn't have to actually drive through Boscastle itself as the road we travelled on came out at the top of Boscastle.

After we had been at home for around a couple of hours, our telephone rang. It was Heather's mother Pat, who asked if we had seen the television news concerning Boscastle. We hadn't and Pat said that we should do so immediately. On went the television and to our horror we saw that Boscastle was being flooded as we could never have even imagined. The police, fire fighters, ambulances and helicopters were shown trying to evacuate the people living there, who were literally trapped in their houses and shops due to the horrendous amount of water flooding the whole village from the car park right through to the harbour (see plates section figures 43-46).

After leaving the hotel I tried to start up a business transfer agency, which is basically an estate agency that sells businesses rather than houses. I set this up whilst at Westcote, the house we had kept after selling the hotel. I managed to secure the prospective sale of three businesses, managing to sell one of them, a restaurant based in Babbacombe, Torquay. Unfortunately I was unable to secure the sale of the others and duly ended the attempt in disappointment. During 2004 whilst living at our new home in Trethevy, a vacancy for a sales representative occurred at Bude Windows & Conservatories. I arranged an interview with the owner, who informed me that he was going to create a new venture in the near future, whereby they would be opening up a new builder's merchants in Bude. It was intended to include the existing manufacturing of their PVC range at the new premises, but he was looking a few months in the future. He informed me that he would contact me again in the future concerning it but for now there was no immediate position available.

During this time Heather was working at a gift shop in Tintagel called The Cats Whiskers as a sales assistant. During the summer months another gift shop called Celtic Legend was advertised for sale. Now this shop was considered by most, including Heather and I, to be the best gift shop in the village. It was owned by a couple called Bill and Patricia Dixon, and we used to frequent the shop occasionally when the situation arose. The stock held was quite superior in quality to most of the others in Tintagel. Both Heather and I had mentioned previously about the possibility of owning a business once again, and this was perhaps a good opportunity of doing so.

Unbeknown to Heather I arranged a viewing with the owners and subject to Heather's agreement informed them that we would make an offer for the business. The shop was situated on the ground floor and had two separate flats above it. One immediately above the shop and the other above that one, in the roof space. The options for the sale of the premises, was split into three parts. This comprised of a) the shop, b) the flat above the shop and c) the flat in the roof space. All were priced separately but if someone wished to buy all three they could do so but any one of the three also. We knew that we could not afford all three but living in Trethevy we quite happy purchasing the shop only. Bill and Trish were happy to sell the shop only, and after our offer had been accepted they decided to keep the flats as residential letting accommodation. After the purchase was completed, again with the assistance of Malcolm Tracey of Eaton Smith and Lloyds Bank, we took over the helm of Celtic Legend on 26th November 2004, which incidentally coincides with Heather's birthday. At the time of writing we are still business partners in Celtic Legend and are now in our sixteenth year of ownership.

Our youngest daughter, Nicola, continued to live with us during this time and quite often assisted in the shop when education permitted. After leaving school at Sir James Smith's in Camelford she attended University in Plymouth, staying in accommodation along with others close to the university, returning home at weekends. In 2008 Heather was returning to thinking of us buying another hotel and Nicola suggested that rather than us stepping straight in and buying one, Heather should perhaps try working in one first in order to make sure of her recent thoughts. A very good suggestion by Nicola, and it wasn't long after that Heather saw an advertisement for a hotel manager in Boscastle which was less than two miles from where we were living in Trethevy. The hotel was called the Bottreaux Hotel and this was a hotel that we had both considered buying shortly after we had sold the Bossiney House Hotel!

At that time it was owned by a man called Graham Mee and it was during February 2002 that it first took our interest. He was actually on holiday in Spain when we first enquired and the lady looking after it in his absence arranged for us to view it, with his permission, of course. We had mixed feelings with it but our main concern was with the central heating system, which we considered to be extremely old and somewhat of a relic, so to speak. However, we did request to see a copy of the hotel's recent accounts and the housekeeper said that she would inform Mr Mee of our request in due course. A few days later a copy of the year 2000's accounts arrived in the mail and Mr Mee informed us that he was returning to Boscastle later that week and invited us to meet him at the hotel in order to discuss things further. The meeting duly took place, and we looked at and inspected the hotel in more detail. We expressed our concern at the apparent state of the heating system, but he stated that it was fine and had never caused him trouble or concern. We then turned our attention to the accounts, the hotel's opening periods and the running of it, etc. This turned out to be somewhat of a complete surprise. We were informed that the hotel was open for business from mid February to the end of October each year and was closed for business between those dates. He then hit us with somewhat of a complete bombshell by informing us that he opened the hotel over Christmas and New Year to guests. He also informed us that the income generated formed quite a substantial amount towards the running of the hotel. That was enough to confirm that our interest in the business was no longer and we informed him as such and left as we had no intentions to work over that period.

Somewhat unbelievably, a few days later we received a letter from him containing an invoice made out to us in respect of his flight costs and time spent in returning from his holiday in Spain and returning to it again! Needless to say we informed him where to get off – so to speak!

He did sell the hotel shortly afterwards and I understand that the new owner apparently made quite a lot of money out of it during 2004/5, following the Boscastle flooding of August 2004. The hotel, being at the top of Boscastle, was completely unaffected by the flooding, whereas the hotels in the bottom of the village were completely closed for weeks afterwards. I think it was in 2006 that the hotel changed hands again to the present owner of the premises.

Heather followed Nicola's suggestion and applied for the position of manager at the Bottreaux, attended an interview with the current owner and was duly offered the position with an almost immediate commencement date. The current manager was a South African lady and she had given notice of termination a week or two previously, as she had decided to return to South Africa. Heather duly commenced employment, with the current manager showing her the way she had been operating the business. Heather immediately realised that the hotel required to be operated in a very different way, as it was quite run down and quiet. It also became obvious that the previous manager had been closing the hotel quite frequently, apparently without the owner, John Acornley, who was based in the midlands, knowing that. A few weeks later, Heather took sole command and took steps to overturn the previous misgivings.

When guests were staying at the hotel, Heather was obviously also expected to stay there in the manager's flat overnight on all occasions. If, however, there were no guests she was able to return to our home in Trethevy overnight, returning to the hotel each day to continue her management duties. It was also stated by the owner that I was allowed to stay with her at the hotel overnight whenever we wished. The hotel was open upon a seasonal basis, and when the season finished and the hotel closed for the winter, Heather returned home more or less full time, visiting the hotel daily in order to check that all was in order, reply to any enquiries and check the mail, etc. I was naturally working at the shop in Tintagel each day, with Heather occasionally joining me there. During the year trade picked up, but it was soon to close for the winter period as in previous years.

The new season started in March 2009 and the hotel became quite busy, and Heather found herself needing to stay overnight in the manager's flat very often. Foolishly I was somewhat reluctant (and stupid, I now realise) to stay every night at the hotel with her and made excuses to stay at our house in Trethevy rather than the hotel. Heather took exception to this, saying that I was no longer interested in her and did not care about her or love her. She told me time and again that she cried herself to sleep being on her own. To this day I am still ashamed of my attitude at the time; it really was unforgivable. Heather was doing a brilliant job there and I told her so regularly. At the end of the season the hotel closed as usual and we both returned to our home in Trethevy. Things were quite strained at times, but our relationship seemed to be getting back to normal during this winter period. We booked a two-week holiday in Lanzarote, staying at the Lanzarote Princess Hotel very close to the sea front. It was unfortunately over much too quickly but nothing untoward was mentioned by either of us about the season before.

During the winter of 2009/10, Heather suggested to the owner that the hotel restaurant and bar, which had been closed for a couple of years or so, be re-opened not only to hotel guests but also non-residents. Obviously, the bar could not be used as a public house but it was perfectly legal for it to be used by diners in the restaurant. I offered to run the bar each evening after being at the shop in order to save wages, as we knew it would not be busy enough to employ someone for quite a while. Heather advertised for a chef/cook to prepare the restaurant meals, we set about preparing the bar and seating area to be ready for guests, ordered the stock of wines and spirits, and it wasn't long before it was ready to go! The chef employed was called Hilary and had previously been chef at the Riverside Restaurant in Boscastle. In addition to the preparation and cooking of the restaurant meals, she also insisted that she would be able to actually serve the meals to the guests. It didn't take long for this part to become obvious that it wasn't possible. Heather and occasionally our youngest daughter, Nicola, took this part over. Breakfasts were prepared by Kim, who had been employed there for some time, as normal. Kim was also housekeeper and was employed almost full time during the season and paid a retainer during winter when the hotel was closed.

This time I was staying at the hotel every night from late February when the hotel re-opened!

In May 2010 a couple of friends from Germany, Klaus and Manu Freitag, along with one of their friends, Ulrike, booked to stay at the hotel for around two weeks. They arrived as planned and seemed to enjoy themselves very much. Klaus was a tour guide with Wikinger Reisen, the German company that we used to deal with at the Bossiney House Hotel. Klaus used to come there for at least one tour, and sometimes two each year. He was also the guide for the special "Bollwein" tour of 1999. They had been staying there for about four days when Heather accused me of telling them in the bar that evening that I was very upset at "having to work in the bar as well as the shop every day" and going on to tell me that Ulrike was particularly adamant that this was wrong of her to expect. To this day I deny that I have ever said that to anyone. I have said to John Acornley on more than one occasion that I only worked in the bar on a night because I loved Heather and that I would not do it otherwise. I believe that that was what was said to Klaus, Manu and Ulrike. That night Heather told me that she wanted us to separate completely at the end of the season, saying that I had upset her so much during the previous season by not staying over and reiterating her feelings towards me. Over the next few days nothing more was said about it and I thought it best not to confront Klaus regarding the matter. However, on the day of their departure, Ulrike had another go at Heather over the matter but this time in a much sterner manner, so Heather informed me. Heather finished up crying over the situation and Klaus has informed me since that he thought that she was crying because they were leaving as their holiday was over and they were going back to Germany.

Most distressingly the situation between us did not improve much, even though I continued staying at the hotel with Heather, sleeping in the same bed almost every night. Every time we tried to talk about it she was so adamant that we should separate that I found myself giving up and agreeing with her. Towards the end of September she insisted that I move out and go back to the house in Trethevy. She also told me that she would look after the bar herself until the end of the season at the end of October. I left thinking and hoping that it would all blow over – how mistaken I was.

For the next few months, although we saw and spoke to each other regularly we remained apart. I was at our home in Trethevy, alone except for our Olly, our Cavalier King Charles Spaniel, and Heather at the Bottreaux. We did spend Christmas Day and Boxing Day 2010 together with family, but not the nights.

Nicola, who had been living at the house with me, decided a few weeks earlier to rent her own home. The house she chose was in Weeks Rise, Camelford, which was approximately fifteen minutes' drive away. She moved into it during August 2010, hence I was now living alone. On New Years Eve the year before, in 2009, she met a young man called Matthew Stedman and they had been going out together as a couple since then. In February 2011 Matthew moved in with Nicola and they have been together ever since. In June 2012 Nicola gave birth to their first son, whom they named Noah. They remained at the house in Weeks Rise for the next couple of years or so, but in 2015 decided to purchase their own home which was situated in Maple Avenue, Camelford, where they remain today. Prior to moving in there during December of that year, they spent a few months living with me at a house I had rented in Otterham, a village near Camelford, following the sale of the house at Trethevy in January 2014. They now have a second son, Elias, who was born in February 2016.

In January 2011 I drove Heather's parents to Bristol Airport in order for them to go on holiday to Portugal, which they had done for a number of years previously. Within a short while of my return home, Heather arrived with a very stern look on her face. She told me that she had something to tell me that was going to upset me a lot. She then informed me that she was having an intimate relationship with John Acornley, the owner of the hotel. Apparently, he had left his wife the previous September, having had enough of their marriage. Naturally I asked her if they were living together and having a sexual relationship, to which she said that had only had sex recently – how recent she would not say. We did have words about the matter and also with John Acornley shortly afterwards, but the words with him will remain untold. Over the next two or three years I could not bring myself to speak to him at all. Things changed when Daniel's father Colin passed away in 2017. At the funeral, John and I were the last two mourners to go into the crematorium, and at the doorway, as we were going in, I offered to call a truce between us. We have been quite okay with each other ever since. Time helps to heal.

In March 2011, I decided to divorce Heather and duly appointed MacMillans Solicitors of Wadebridge to act upon my behalf. In September 2012 our divorce was finalised and our marriage of thirty-four years (thirty-two actually together) was over. Heather and John tied the knot together by getting married in May 2014. Heather and I soon became good friends again because after all, we had been married for a long time, had two children together and, of course, now five grandchildren, not to mention the shop in Tintagel - Celtic Legend.

During 2010 I had been experiencing slight problems when swallowing food, which was occasionally seeming to get a little stuck in my throat. I quite often had to swallow water in order to clear it but didn't think that it was anything serious enough to obtain medical advice. This continued for the next couple of years pretty much in the same way. However, towards the end of August 2012 it seemed to be getting worse, so I arranged an appointment with my GP, Dr Graham Garrod, at Tintagel Surgery, who suggested that further medical advice should be sought from a throat specialist. On 5th October I was examined at Bodmin Hospital by an endoscopist, Mr Ruseckas, who diagnosed that a pharyngeal pouch was probably the cause of my problem. On Monday 19th November I attended an examination at the screening department at the Royal Cornwall Hospital in Truro, whereby it was confirmed that I did indeed have a pharyngeal pouch in the back of my throat that would require surgery in order to repair. An appointment was duly made and the operation finally took place on 13th February 2013. I was operated upon during the afternoon, kept in overnight and Heather, who very kindly drove me there, picked me up the following afternoon and drove me back to the house in Trethevy. Thankfully the problem has not occurred again and hopefully will not do so.

The house at Trethevy was finally sold in January 2014 and the vast majority of the proceeds went straight to Lloyds Bank Ltd, with the balance being split between Heather and myself. The reason for the Lloyds Bank involvement was due to the financial recession of 2008/9, whereby the sales at the shop dropped absolutely dramatically almost overnight. From being a very good, profitable, self-supporting business, we were plunged into a financial nightmare. In order to buy the shop in the first place, we had borrowed a substantial amount from Lloyds. After the recession hit we finished up having to arrange overdraft facilities in order to help pay the business loan monthly instalments in addition to paying suppliers for stock. Without the stock there would be nothing to sell in order to keep things going at all. We still have the shop together but that is up for sale as well. Unfortunately, if that is the right word, since the recession hit us in 2008/9 we have had to endure the Brexit referendum of 2016, which affected business quite dramatically, followed by the currently ongoing coronavirus pandemic, which has caused the complete closure of all non-essential shops although it is, hopefully, for a temporary unknown period of time. In effect the turnover of the business has reduced by approximately sixty-five per cent since we bought it in November 2004 to date.

Following our divorce and the eventual sale of the house in January 2014, I have lived in rented accommodation due to the obvious financial restrictions. From the house in Trethevy I moved to a bungalow in Otterham, Camelford, where I stayed until September 2016. In early 2015 Nicola, Matthew and Noah decided to try and purchase their own home, and asked me if they could move in with me at the bungalow I was renting at the time, in order to save money on renting whilst they were looking around to buy their own first home together. After asking permission from the owner of the bungalow I was renting, they moved in with me. The bungalow had three bedrooms but I was using one of them, the smallest, as an office, as I have always attended to the shop accounts at home rather than in the shop itself for obvious reasons. They consequently moved in using the spare bedroom, which was already set up with a double bed, etc., and Noah's cot fitted in quite snugly as well. It was quite a good arrangement for them, saved them a bit of cash which went towards their forthcoming purchase, and was also good for me in more ways than one!

In July of that year, I started getting what I can only describe as gradual blindness in my left eye. It started with an area at the bottom right, gradually getting darker and darker, like a black shadow growing larger by the day. A couple of days later, on 9th July, I could hardly see out of my left eye at all and made an emergency appointment with my new doctor, who was taking over as my personal doctor from Dr Garrod, who was in the course of retiring from the practice. She asked me a few questions as to what was the apparent problem, said that it was too light in the surgery to examine the eye properly and then diagnosed that I had experienced a second stroke. I insisted that her diagnosis was wrong and that the problem was directly an eye problem. She was absolutely adamant that the problem was a stroke and that she would contact the Royal Cornwall Hospital in Truro by email that afternoon in order for them to arrange an appointment for me to see them.

The following afternoon, Friday 10th July, I was contacted by the hospital and was offered an examination either at Truro the following day or the following Tuesday at Bodmin, which was more local. As the doctor had informed me that I could no longer drive until the problem was sorted, I initially informed them I would take the Bodmin appointment. I then rang Nicola from the shop to tell her what had happened and ask her to pick me up, as I could no longer drive myself. Two minutes later she rang back, told me in no uncertain terms to immediately contact the Hospital in Truro and rearrange the appointment to Saturday 11th July, and that she, Matthew and Noah would take me there and of course take me back home again. They duly drove me to the Royal Hospital the following day. I was thoroughly examined by a couple of nurses and, not to my surprise, informed that I had definitely not had a stroke and that the problem was an eye problem that required immediate attention. The ward nurse rang the ophthalmology department and I was requested to report there for examination. After waiting approximately a further three hours in that department, that was extremely busy with patients, I was examined by a consultant, a Mr George, who informed me that I had a left eye retinal detachment that required an immediate operation. I was asked to wait until he had managed to have a word with an eye surgeon, Mr Murjaneh, who was currently in the operating theatre. The outcome an hour or so later was an operation arranged for the following morning. Nicola and family picked me up, and took me back to the bungalow for the night. Nicola then drove me back to the hospital again for 8.00am the following morning, and after being examined by the surgeon, Mr Murjaneh, he was operating on me by 9.00am. The consent form completed by Mr George referred to my right eye not the left; this I pointed out to Mr Murjaneh that morning. Well, mistakes do happen occasionally. It was then back home with various medications, instructions on how to sleep, how to hold my head whilst awake, how to lie down during the day for forty-five minutes at a time on my right hand side only, with a fifteen-minute "toilet break" before lying down again – then repeat it all for the rest of the day! This I had to do repeatedly for six weeks with occasional hospital visits in between.

On 23rd July I decided to write a letter to Dr Garrod outlining the problems I had incurred and the lead-up to them concerning the diagnosis by the doctor previously.

A few days later I received a reply from Dr Radford dated 29th July informing me that my letter would be shared and reviewed at the clinical team meeting to be held shortly. A further letter from Drs Garrod and Abbott dated 4th August was received informing me of the outcome of that meeting (see plates section figures 48-49).

Nicola, Matthew and Noah were looking after me very attentively and it was very much as well that they were living with me at the bungalow. If I had been there alone, who knows what might have been. Every day my medicine and eye drops were prepared and administered by Nicola with Noah in close attendance. They bought me a small kitchen timer which when set alerted me to the timings required for my new daily routine. Nicola made all of our meals, looked after the house as well as me, Matthew attended to the garden, etc., and Noah was always in attendance doing as much as he could for me. Pat and John, Heather's parents, occasionally drove me to the hospital and back again on the days that appointments had been made for my regular check-ups. This routine went on for the next six weeks and I was requested to attend the hospital on Wednesday 19th August at 2.00pm for my final check-up and probable discharge. However, when I awoke on the morning of 17th August, I realised that I was once again experiencing the same problem in my left eye. This time the dark patches were commencing at the top left of my eye. Nicola immediately rang the hospital and I was advised to attend immediately. Nicola once again drove me there and back again, of course. Following this examination I was given an appointment for a second operation for 8.00am the following morning, 18th August. Once again in for an operation but this time the detachment was at the top of my eye, directly opposite the first detachment. Another six weeks of the same treatment and medication, but this time my forty-five minutes of lying down had to be on my left hand side only. The lying down was required for the gas that was injected into my eye, to "float" over the operated area of my retina, therefore keeping the intraocular pressure controlled in order for the repair to be successful.

Once again it was Nicola, Matthew and Noah to the rescue for the six-week period, with Pat and John chauffeuring me to and from the hospital as required. Eventually I was given the all-clear with the exception of being informed that I would require cataract surgery and implant on my left eye once the retinal operation had settled down. This eventually took place on 22nd February 2016 at 2.15pm. Following a final check-up on 25th May 2016 I was informed that all was now well, but that I would probably require cataract surgery on my right eye sometime in the future. Somewhat of a traumatic time for me, and my thanks go to the hospital teams and, of course, Nicola, Matthew, Noah, Pat and John for the much-valued help and assistance.

Nicola and family succeeded in purchasing their first home together and moved into it just before Christmas 2015. The house was a three-bedroom property in Maple Avenue, Camelford, where they still live today. They can't get away from me, though, as I now rent a property next door to them! More of this later.

A few months after they moved into their new home, Matthew informed me that he had seen the bungalow at Otterham in the houses for sale column in the local newspaper. To say that I was taken by surprise is an understatement. I immediately looked at the Rightmove website and there it was advertised as plain as day. The owner, who had lived in another bungalow that he owned next door to me but had recently sold it and moved to St Columb, had not had the decency to say a word to me about it. The bungalow had apparently been on the market for some fifteen months! So I decided to look for alternative accommodation.

During December 2015 and January 2016 we had experienced extremely high winds which had caused quite a bit of damage around the area, particularly to trees and fences, etc. Damage to the fences around the gardens and a fallen tree were reported by me to him and he informed me that he would come and have a look around. During the Christmas break the boiler would not work. I rang him and he asked me to ring Steve Goodman, a plumbing and heating engineer from Tintagel, for advice on the problem. Steve advised me to check the cut-off valve, which I did as we were still on the telephone to each other. That was apparently the problem and it was working again. Steve also advised me to request the owner to arrange for the boiler to be serviced sooner rather than later. This I did, but to no avail.

Early in April I tried to contact the owner again as the oil tank that supplied the boiler for the heating and hot water had developed a fault and oil was not getting to the boiler. When I eventually managed to contact him, he informed me that he was away in Preston, Lancashire, and that if there was a problem with the boiler I would have to sort it out myself. With no heating and no hot water (the immersion heater had never worked – which he knew about), I had no option but to contact a local plumber, Brian Faulkner, who lived in Boscastle. With the weather being so bad he was quite busy, but he inspected the tank within a couple of days. The outcome was that the tank required a replacement oil valve for the existing one that was excessively corroded and therefore solid and a sight glass that was broken and also unreadable through age. The approximate cost would be £95.00, but the job could not be done for a few days as the parts required ordering and he was also extremely busy with other jobs. It was nine days before he was able to return and complete the work. I was therefore another nine days without heating or hot water. He also said that the boiler badly needed servicing and I duly informed the owner as such.

When I first agreed to take up the rental, a number of things throughout the bungalow that required attention were agreed to be either repaired, replaced or removed at his expense and doing. Amongst the things requiring attention were: replacement glazing of the patio doors leading out of the dining room to the rear garden, replacement glazing in windows in the bedrooms and lounge, bedroom window framework and beading, removal of the Porsche car in the garage, removal of the three cars in the bungalow driveway, removal of various rubbish in the lane immediately outside the driveway entrance, the emptying of the greenhouse and the garden shed, and replacement of the immersion heater. The Porsche was eventually removed in April, and whilst two of the cars in the driveway were eventually removed, one of the cars was still parked there when I left the bungalow in September 2016. It was still there when the bungalow was eventually sold to a Mr and Mrs Neate some months later.

On 23rd August 2016 I wrote to him and his partner, giving them one month's notice of my intention to leave. Prior to the letter I informed them verbally by telephone and they actually refused to give me their new address of which to send the official letter of termination. I was informed by them that their reason for refusal was so that I would be unable to divulge their new address to others! Within the letter I included the reasons for my decision along with a breakdown of costs borne by myself that would be deducted from my final months rent. Effectively he received a final payment of £406.21 as opposed to the full month's rent of £700.00. The damage caused by the winds as stated above had still not been touched by him at the time of my departure. The tree that been blown down was partially removed by the next-door neighbour and the other part being left embedded in the greenhouse.

Shortly afterwards I received a telephone call asking me to reconsider my decision to leave, along with him promising to take the bungalow off the market and guarantee that they would not try to sell it for another three years. The man must have thought that I was born the day before or that I was some sort of idiot! During my tenure I had paid him £22,400.00 in monthly rent and he had spent NOTHING on the bungalow whatsoever, except for perhaps the building's insurance! When I left in September 2016 the greenhouse and shed were still full of the things he had put in there and the boiler still hadn't been serviced.

Then it was to a converted barn at Halgabron, Tintagel, that was owned by Margaret and Philip Nute, a local farming family that we had known since coming to live in Cornwall in 1996. The barn was situated in the farm grounds and the milking sheds were only a few yards away. It was a three-bedroom property and initially was very comfortable in which to live. I moved in there in September 2016 and found the property to be nice and warm. However, when the winter arrived I found it to be very cold there as the heating system comprised of night storage heaters, two of which were in the lounge and one in each of the dining room, the three bedrooms, bathroom and landing. Unfortunately they were all very old, two of which were dated 1990. No matter how they were set by the time I arrived home at the end of the day there was very little heat left in them. Even though I purchased an electric heater, which was very good and efficient, it wasn't enough to keep sufficiently warm. I decided to look elsewhere and Nicola mentioned a house in Camelford that was becoming available literally next door to them. After viewing it, although the rental was more than I had been paying, I decided to take it. I had a chat with Margaret and informed her as to why I had made the decision to move. She was very understanding and a couple of days later informed me that due to my main reason being the heating system, they had decided to have an oil heated central heating system installed throughout. Being part of the farm, so to speak, there was also concern over the obvious flies that were around almost all of the time. Where there are cows there are flies. They were not in the house itself much at all, but where my car was parked under the car port, there were literally hundreds of them day and night. My light blue Ford Focus was permanently littered with fly spots of you know what, all over the bodywork.

I took the lease on for the house in Maple Avenue, from 1st February 2017, although I didn't actually move in until late February. It is a four-bedroom property linked to Nicola and Matthew's house by the garage at one side and partially at the other side next-door neighbour's by part of the house itself. It has three upstairs bedrooms, one with en-suite which I use, the smallest of which is used as a dressing room, the other being set up as a spare bedroom and a house bathroom. Downstairs is bedroom four, which I use as an office, a lounge, a dining room, a large kitchen, a downstairs toilet and garage. The house has oil-fired central heating and is very comfortable. I just hope that the current owner doesn't decide sell it! Not whilst I am here anyway.

Having moved from the house at Halgabron, I informed the doctorate at Tintagel of my change of address, verbally with Linda the receptionist at the surgery. On 2nd March I received a letter from the practice business manager, informing me that I could no longer remain as a patient with the practice as I no longer resided in their core catchment area. He informed me of the available doctors situated in Camelford and suggested I register with one of them. He did state within his letter that I could appeal the decision by writing to the Bottreaux Surgery in Boscastle, which I did that same day. I eventually received a reply from him within a letter dated 20th March informing me that my appeal had been rejected by the partners, one of whom was his wife – the doctor who diagnosed my "stroke" in 2015. I have often wondered whether or not my letter to Dr Graham Garrod, a partner in the practice at the time, outlining my appointment with his colleague, may have had a bearing on the resulting outcome of my rejection and subsequent appeal. I sometimes still do.

It has been very good for me being next door to Nicola and family, especially as I get to see them all regularly without living in each other's pocket, so to speak. As I mentioned briefly beforehand, Nicola's youngest son Elias was born on 25th February 2016 and his pending birth was another of their reasons for wanting to buy their own home. Having moved in during the previous December, it was perfect timing for the arrival of Elias. With me moving in next door the following year, I have been very fortunate to see both Noah and Elias growing up and them very gradually getting to know life. I had the fortune to babysit occasionally, and for a while in late 2018 and early 2019 sat for them almost every Thursday evening while Nicola and Matthew spent about an hour at a local keep-fit club. It was shortly to become even more important for me to be living close at hand.

In October 2018 I developed an excruciating pain in my lower back area. A friend of mine who lived in Brighouse suggested that it may be sciatica, which she had experienced recently. It gradually got worse, and at the beginning of November I decided to make an appointment with my doctor, who was now situated in Camelford with me having moved away from the Tintagel area. My new doctor asked me what my symptoms were and I explained the area and type of pain I was experiencing and that it had been suggested by a friend to be sciatica. He duly agreed that could be the problem but without examining me at all other than taking my blood pressure. He informed me that he would issue a prescription for a course of painkillers and that if the symptoms were still prevalent in two weeks' time, I should contact a physiotherapist and arrange for further treatment. The two weeks went by without any improvement whatsoever and I contacted one of the physiotherapists that had been recommended by my doctor. Following an examination he informed me that it was not sciatica but a twisted pelvis that was the problem. He was certain that was the problem and gave me a series of exercises to do for the next week before returning for a second examination. A second examination, a couple of exercises and some heat treatment followed, and a third appointment made with exercises for another week. I attended once again for the same treatment to be given and an appointment for a fourth time. The physiotherapist informed me that the fourth course of treatment would be the last one that could be paid for by the NHS and that any further treatment after that would have to be paid for by myself.

I agreed to return the following week but decided to also arrange for an examination by an osteopath who had a practice at Wainhouse Corner on the A38 near Bude and had been recommended to me. At the appointment she asked me various questions, gave me an initial examination and duly informed me that both the doctor and physiotherapist were wrong with their diagnosis, and I had in fact got torn muscles in my thighs. That cost me about £50.00 for about thirty minutes but I made a second appointment with her for two weeks later. I attended my fourth appointment with the physiotherapist but did not arrange any more. After attending the second one with the osteopath, and another £40.00, I decided enough was enough and to leave things for a while and see how they developed. Over Christmas and the New Year the problem didn't feel any better but didn't any worse either, but I had also developed a really bad cold. I was coughing somewhat excessively particularly overnight. With the time of year the doctor's surgery was closed, of course, and I decided to call for help by dialling 111. After explaining what was wrong with me the operator informed me that she would arrange for a doctor to call me. Within five minutes I received the call back and was advised to take paracetamol tablets and drink plenty of water. If things hadn't improved in two or three days, contact my doctor and arrange an appointment.

Fortunately things did improve from that point of view but the back pain was as bad as ever. In mid January I decided to contact my doctor and request for an X-ray to be taken, as I was convinced that something was very wrong with me. The doctor arranged for the X-ray to be taken at Bodmin Hospital on 24th January, which I attended with some relief. I was informed that the results would be sent to my doctor within the next few days. On 4th February I received a letter dated 30th January (posted second class), requesting me to contact the surgery to arrange an appointment to see the doctor regarding the result of my recent X-ray. I saw my doctor the following day and was informed that the X-ray revealed that my left hip needed replacing due to severe arthritis. The letter also inferred that my right hip may also require replacing but was not as bad as the left one. He then informed me that he would send a letter to the Cornwall Referral Management Service requesting that an operation be granted. In the meantime I was prescribed a stronger painkiller. On 15th February I received a letter from the medical secretary at Camelford Surgery that was dated 11th February (posted second class) informing me that, "You recently visited your GP at the surgery who referred you to see a specialist with regard to further care, advice or treatment. We have been informed by the Referral Management Service that your referral has been rejected. If you wish to discuss this further please contact the surgery and make an appointment to see the doctor."

Obviously this decision came as something of a bombshell and I immediately rang the surgery for an appointment to see the doctor. At the appointment I asked him why the referral had been rejected and he didn't seem to know that it had. He referred to his notes via his computer and his reply was that, "It would appear that we did not supply them with sufficient information." He then informed me that he would send in another application containing all the information they had. This, I presume, meant enclosing a copy of the X-ray detailing the hip problems and the physiotherapist's reports from December. A few days later, I was informed that the second application had been accepted, and that I would be hearing directly from the NHS with regard to further information. On 26th February I did indeed receive a telephone call at the shop, in order to arrange an appointment to see a specialist. They offered me appointments at three different hospitals with dates ranging from March through to June. I elected to see a specialist at the Peninsular NHS Treatment Centre in Plymouth on Tuesday 12th March at 11.50am. This was the earliest appointment available and I was very happy to accept it. I don't know what I would have been feeling like if the June date had been the earliest available. I received a letter from them confirming the appointment dated 27th February by first class mail!

I do realise how busy doctors can be and that quite a lot of their patients can be very impatient regarding treatment, etc. What I can't understand is why they use second class postage services in situations similar, or perhaps worse than the situation referred to above. It just doesn't seem right to me. If it boils down to the extra cost between first and second class stamps, it amounted to around 8p in February 2019.

On 12th March 2019 I attended as arranged, and after having various examinations for blood pressure, heart rate, breathing, etc., I had another X-ray prior to meeting the surgeon, Mr Wudecki, who showed me the results of the X-rays and went through the various steps in the procedures that would be required. The X-rays of my hips very clearly showed that there was severe osteoarthritis in my left hip, and whilst the right hip was infected with osteoarthritis, it was not as badly infected but would require treatment in the not too distant future. He then completed a "Patient agreement to investigate or treatment" consent form outlining that I would require a replacement left hip, which I had to sign, as did he. When I asked him when my operation might be he told me that there was a very short waiting list at the time, and that it may be within the month, April. That was more or less it for then and all I had to do now was wait for the actual date. I also attended an appointment at the anaesthetist clinic at the same hospital on 21st March at 10.40am, whereby the anaesthetist informed me of what to expect in that respect. All very straightforward, I am glad to say, even though it was another ninety-mile round trip – well worth it.

April arrived and my anticipation levels also arrived, as I was expecting the operation date to arrive any day now. However, towards the end of the month I hadn't heard anything and decided to ring them for further information. The receptionist informed me that no date had been decided upon as yet, but she would ask the operations manager, Chris, to contact me regarding it. Shortly afterwards he did ring me but said that it may be some time yet. When I told him that Mr Wudecki had suggested that it might be in April, he told me that the waiting list was quite a few weeks long. He suggested that I could go on a cancellation list but that might mean short notice. When I mentioned that Mr Wudecki had also suggested this list he seemed surprised. The result was that I was now on that list. Lo and behold, he rang me a few days later to inform me that a cancellation had arisen and would I consider the operation to take place on 10th May. My reply? YES PLEASE! THANK YOU!

I then received a letter from NHS Community Orthopaedic Service Hospital in Liskeard to attend an appointment on 30th April at 11.30am in order to discuss the loan of various support equipment that I might need following the operation. I duly attended and the following week the equipment was delivered to me. It was all very helpful during my recovery and I can't thank them enough for it. The equipment was collected by them and returned in the original packaging some six months later.

On Friday 10th May Nicola drove me to the Peninsular Hospital for my operation. We arrived at around 1.00pm and reported to the reception area, and after waiting for only a few minutes, I was escorted to the operating theatre area waiting room and Nicola returned home. I was then asked to remove all my clothes and put on one of those flimsy operating gowns and to fasten it at the back by tying the cords together. Due to the stroke I suffered all that time ago, I have always had a problem when using my right arm and hand, and couldn't fasten the gown at all. When the nurse returned a few minutes later she fastened it for me and helped place my clothes in a couple of bags. I was then asked to wait there until I was called for my operation. At approximately 4.00pm I was on my way to the operating theatre in a wheelchair. After being briefly examined by Mr Wudecki and the anaesthetist, I was given the anaesthetics required for the operation, being a spinal injection and sedation. The next thing I knew was waking up in the recovery area – operation completed.

A little later I was wheeled to Room 12 in the hospital recuperation ward. Shortly afterwards wheeled again to Room 3, where I stayed for about five minutes before being moved for the third time to Room 1, where I remained until my discharge three days later. The following morning I was advised to keep moving about the room periodically using a walking frame, which was quite tiring, but I did as advised. Just before lunchtime Mr Wudecki came to see me, along with a physiotherapist. They asked me how I was feeling and asked me to walk with the help of the frame in the ward. This I did, but to my utmost surprise Mr Wudecki said that I was fit enough to be discharged and I was asked to arrange to be collected that afternoon. Now, I was expecting to be there for at least three days and Nicola had arranged to come and see me that afternoon, along with Matthew, Noah and Elias. I informed him of this and he said that he would arrange for my discharge papers to be ready later that afternoon and they could drive me home. Shortly after lunchtime Nicola and family arrived and I told them about the decision by Mr Wudecki. They were even more surprised than I was earlier in the day. They asked me how I was managing to walk with the frame and I said that was alright. We carried on talking for a few minutes and I then stood up and walked to the room door and back again, taking my time, of course. I sat back down on my chair and within a few seconds started lose my breath. My chest felt as though it was bursting, and within seconds I was gasping for breath. I honestly thought that I was having a heart attack or something worse. I thought my time was up and I was going to die. I am not exaggerating – it was that bad. Nicola immediately pressed the emergency bell and ran to the door calling out to the nurses for help. In they rushed and immediately put the oxygen mask over my face, but I was panicking like I had never done before. They asked Nicola, Matthew and the boys to wait outside whilst trying to alleviate the problem I was experiencing. I was asked to try to relax and take deep slow breaths of the oxygen in order for my breathing to become natural again. After a few minutes it worked; I started breathing normally, still with the oxygen mask in place, and eventually my body relaxed. Nicola and family were asked to come back in for a while in order for them to see that I was almost back to normal. I know that they feared the worst when it all happened, as did I. After a few minutes they were asked to leave me to fully recover and they made their way back home to Camelford. I remained on the oxygen for a while longer and the nurses kept looking in on me for the rest of the day. I was later told that the problem

I had experienced was down to a very sharp drop in my blood pressure. I have never felt like that before or, thankfully, since. It was the most frightening experience of my life.

Needless to say, it was decided to keep me in overnight under more or less constant supervision.

The following afternoon Laura, Daniel, Sophie and Chloe came to see me, and whilst they were with me I was visited by the ward doctor. After discussing the problem of the day before, in which Laura was very much involved, it was decided to keep me in for at least one more night. On the Monday morning, just before lunchtime, I was visited by the doctor and a couple of physiotherapists. After being asked how I was now feeling, which was much, much better, they suggested that I walk from the ward to the physiotherapy department in order to determine my progress. I was asked to walk up and down a mock staircase, holding on to the banisters for safety, of course, and a physiotherapist behind me, just in case. Back in the ward they gave me a couple of other tests and decided that if I wanted to, and only if I wanted to, I could be discharged. Otherwise I could stay for at least one more night. I elected to be discharged and then rang Nicola to ask her to pick me up and drive me home. When she arrived to collect me, I was wheeled out of the hospital in a wheelchair by a nurse, who then showed me how to get into and out of a vehicle safely without putting excess strain on my new hip.

Prior to going into hospital for the operation, it had been suggested by Nicola and Laura to move my bed from my bedroom upstairs into the dining room downstairs for the duration of my convalescence. When I arrived home it had been moved accordingly with the dining table and chairs now in the kitchen. The equipment supplied to me by the NHS had already been put into the downstairs WC and lounge, etc. I had asked Laura to collect a walking frame that I had ordered from Argos which had been given to Nicola prior to picking me up. All was in place thanks to my wonderful family and the road to recovery was underway.

Every morning at around 7.45am Nicola and Elias used to come in, and Nicola would make me a light breakfast and mug of coffee, and Elias would bring me my morning's dose of medication, four various tablets and a glass of water. They would then return a little later, usually after they had taken Noah to school, and help me with getting dressed and occasionally a few other things that I couldn't manage myself. For example, I had been informed that I should not bend down or lean over to put on my socks, wash my feet or cut my toenails, vacuum the carpets, lift anything even slightly heavy, not to put things into high or low cupboards or drawers, or attempt anything that might cause me to fall over, possibly damaging my new hip. Nicola washed my hair and back and feet whenever required, cooked my meals next door at their house most days, and would bring them round to mine at mealtimes, including lunchtime. Heather would look after my needs at lunchtimes occasionally, and Laura and family cooked my evening meals a few times, usually eating their meals with me at the same time. I was being looked after extremely well. Thanks to all for everything; I certainly could not have managed without them. On 24th May I had the staples removed from my operation incision at the Camelford Surgery. Nicola did notice afterwards that the nurse had accidentally left three of the staples, which they removed a day or so later.

During June I received a letter from Peninsular NHS regarding a post-operative follow-up appointment that had been arranged for 9th July at 11.15am. I duly attended and after a somewhat brief consultation was given the all-clear. A big difference here was that I could officially drive my own car once again – legally. Finally in November I received an "After Your Operation" Questionnaire, which I completed and returned on 28th November. Thankfully all is now well with the new hip and I am no longer in any pain due to it. However, the right hip is steadily reminding me of the problems I experienced beforehand and is possibly beginning to deteriorate in a similar way. I was due to have a twelve-month check-up at the Peninsular sometime during May 2020, but due to the current coronavirus pandemic situation this took place by telephone in December 2020.

Since our separation and divorce I have endured somewhat of a mixed time in my life in one way and another. My youngest brother Glyn unfortunately passed away in January 2014 whilst I was on holiday in the Algarve. My Uncle Arthur (Dad's youngest brother) passed away the following January 2015 (Algarve again), Aunty Muriel (Mum's older sister) in December 2017, John Peaker (football and cricketing colleague and friend) in November 2019, and my cousin Geoff in February 2020. In addition to the above a further six friends from the Tintagel area have passed away.

On a more cheerful note, Glyn's youngest daughter Catherine married in August 2014 and gave birth to a daughter (Erica Rachel) in June 2018; Nicola, her sons Noah in June 2012 and Elias in February 2016; and Laura gave birth to her son Isaac in December 2019.

Although being single once again, I have also enjoyed holidaying in Lanzarote a couple of times and many times in Albufeira in the Algarve. Whilst I would have much preferred to have been accompanied by my ex-wife Heather, I have enjoyed most of the times I have visited the places and making new friends, particularly in Albufeira. Amongst these people I include at Buddy's Bar & Restaurant – Claudia, Vanessa, Marcella, Patricia, Eduardo, Chico and all; Paulu's Pizzeria – Claudia (again), John and all; Wild & Co – Carlos and Nuno; Pratos do Dia – Nuesa; Ouratlantico Apartments - Rui, Christina and all.

All in all, I know that I have had a good life in general without too many setbacks. I have had the odd medical problem in recent years but nothing really substantial, except for possibly the stroke in 1996.

Medical problems:
May 1996 – stroke.
February 2013 – throat operation, pharyngeal pouch.
June 2015 – retinal detachment, left eye.
August 2015 – second detachment, left eye.
May 2019 – left hip, total replacement.
February 2021 – cataract surgery, right eye.

The worst things in my life:
Being separated from and then divorcing Heather.
Starting smoking.
Having a stroke.

The best things in my life:
Marrying Heather.
Having our two children.
Our children having their children (our grandchildren).
Stopping smoking (09.02.86).

Well, I think that that is just about it, but if I have forgotten anything or not mentioned anyone, I apologise. The full content of this autobiography is completely factual and I am not aware of any misgivings within my writings.

List of Figures

13. Learner's swimming certificate, 1961.
14. Flood showing river by Armitage Bridge Church, which is on the left (permission of *Huddersfield Examiner/MEN Media*).
15. Flood showing river near to the church (permission of *Huddersfield Examiner/MEN Media*).
16. Flood showing river from the rookery looking towards the farm (permission of *Huddersfield Examiner/MEN Media*).
17. Newsome Secondary School.
18. Lockwood CYC under-seventeen football team circa 1965/66.

    Back row: Les Clark, unknown, John Copley, David Beaumont, Stephen Goddard, Stephen Fitt, Ian Graham; front row: Kenneth Binns, Michael Drake, unknown, Trevor Manning, Barry Bloy.
19. Hall Bower Cricket Club looking towards Castle Hill.
20. Byrom Shield winners, 1967 – Hall Bower Cricket Club First X1.

    Back row: Peter Thorpe, Harold Bray, Michael Barron, Terry Heaton, Roy MacNairey, Derek Stow, Ian Booth, John Ogden, Ken Graham, Jack McShane (Rackie – Jack's dog); front row: Ian Graham, Geoff Heywood, Tommy Galvin, Barry Robertshaw, Harold Galley.
21. Sykes Cup winners, 1972 – Hall Bower First X1.

    Back row: Stuart Greaves, Ian Booth, Terry Woodhouse, John Peaker, Stephen Lawrence; front row: Barry Robertshaw, Ian Graham, Robert Moorhouse, Geoff Heywood, Peter Ramsden, John Greaves.
22. Paddock Shield winners, 1977 – Hall Bower Second X1.
23. Match report, Paddock Shield Final (permission of *Huddersfield Examiner/MEN Media*).
24. Pantomime cast during finale of "Old King Cole" in 1967 (permission of *Huddersfield Examiner/MEN Media*).
25. Pantomime – report of presentation of *Cinderella* in 1965 (permission of *Huddersfield Examiner/MEN Media*).
26. Staff changes, Hepworth Iron Company, 1987.
27. Letter from Raymond Hirst.
28. Letter to Mrs Hirst.
29. Letter from Mrs Hirst.
30. Samson Lintels, change of management.
31. Eaton Smith & Downey, Bankfield Park House costs.
32. Bankfield Park Avenue just after purchased in 1978.